C. Boutin J. R. Viallat Y. Aelony

Practical Thoracoscopy

With the Collaboration of F. Rey

Foreword by R. W. Light

With 70 Figures (46 in color) and 13 Tables

Springer-Verlag
Berlin Heidelberg New York London
Paris Tokyo Hong Kong Barcelona

Professor Dr. CHRISTIAN BOUTIN
Hopital de la Conception, 147 Bd. Baille
13385 Marseille Cedex 5, France

JEAN RÉGIS VIALLAT, MD
Department of Pneumology
Paoli-Calmettes Institute
13009 Marseilles, France

YOSSEF AELONY, MD
Department of Internal Medicine and Pulmonology
Southern California Permanente Medical Group
Harbor City, CA 90710, USA

1st edition 1991
2nd printing 1992

ISBN 3-540-52369-3 Springer-Verlag Berlin Heidelberg New York
ISBN 0-387-52369-3 Springer-Verlag New York Berlin Heidelberg

Library of Congress Cataloging-in-Publication Data
Boutin, C. (Christian), 1933- Practical thoracoscopy / C. Boutin, J. R. Viallat, Y. Aelony ; with collaboration of F. Rey; foreword by R. W. Light. Includes bibliographical references and index. ISBN 3-540-52369-3 Springer-Verlag Berlin Heidelberg New York. - ISBN 0-387-52369-3 Springer-Verlag New York Berlin Heidelberg 1. Thoracoscopy. I. Viallat, J. R. (Jean Régis), 1947-. II. Aelony, Y. (Yossef), 1939-. III. Title. RC941.B 68 1991 617.5′407545--dc20

Typesetting, printing and binding: Appl, Wemding
23/3145-54321 - Printed on acid-free paper

Foreword

Diseases of the pleura such as effusion, thickening, or pneumothorax are frequently encountered in the practice of medicine. *Practical Thoracoscopy* presents an encyclopedic approach to the use of thoracoscopy in the diagnosis and treatment of patients with pleural disease.

After an initial chapter on the history of thoracoscopy, the next three chapters of the book are devoted to the general technique of performing thoracoscopy, a topic on which the team of Dr. Boutin and his colleagues write with ample experience. In these chapters they provide detailed descriptions of how to perform the procedure and discuss the pros and the cons of the different approaches and the different equipment available. The following chapter discusses the complications of the procedure.

The next chapter discusses the role of thoracoscopy in diagnosing pleural effusions. My own opinion here is in general that, as long as well trained personnel are available, thoracoscopy is preferable to open pleural biopsy, because it is associated with less morbidity and mortality and can be done if necessary under local anesthesia.

The following chapter is directed at using to thoracoscopy to facilitate pleurodesis for chronic pleural effusions. With Boutin's method, talc poudrage is performed during thoracoscopy, and certainly, if a thoracoscopy is used to establish the diagnosis of a malignant pleural effusion, it is appropriate to attempt to induce a pleurodesis with talc at the time of the diagnostic procedure.

The next chapter discusses the role of thoracoscopy in the management of patients with pneumothorax. It is likely that thoracoscopy will in future achieve a greater role in managing spontaneous pneumothorax if it is shown that laser therapy or therapy with fibrin glue through the thoracoscope is useful in closing bronchopleural fistulas.

Practical Thoracoscopy is a very practical book by one of the world's authorities on thoracoscopy. This book is recommended for those individuals who are presently doing the procedure or plan to learn the procedure in the future. It will also be useful to pulmonary subspecialists who wish to learn more about thoracoscopy.

Autumn 1990

Richard W. Light
Long Beach, Calif.

Acknowledgments

This book is the result of long collaboration by all of the members of our medical team. I would especially like to thank all of those who have contributed to perfecting the method: Paul Cargnino, who began with me over 20 years ago, and Paulette Farisse, who is a tireless collaborator. Professor Jacques Farisse has greatly increased our knowledge of pleural anatomy and we are very grateful; thanks to him, we have been able to organize thoracoscopy courses at the Marseilles School of Medicine. We are grateful to Annie Martin for her abilities in anesthesiology; thanks to her, all of our patients have undergone examinations in comfort. We would also like to thank all of the assistants who have worked in the department: Michel Irisson, Jean-Marc Velardocchio, Hervé Jullian, Hervé Le Caer, Ghislaine Convert, Philippe Astoul, Bernard Seitz, and Jean-Louis Fico.

We would especially like to thank Peter Tucker for his help with the English version of this book.

Finally, we thank our secretaries for their very great patience: Martine Roure, Elisabeth Eynier, Martine Veropalumbo, Marie-Pierre Pignolo, and Marie-Françoise Riot.

This book could never have been written without the help of the Richard Wolf GmbH. The understanding and abilities of Messrs. Hildebrandt and Heckele have enabled us, since 1976, constantly to improve our equipment.

Contents

Introduction

Thousands of thoracoscopies were carried out for the lysis of pleural adhesions (pneumonolysis) between 1910, the year the technique was invented by the Swede Jacobaeus, and 1950–1955 when it became obsolete following the discovery of antituberculous drugs. These thoracoscopies were carried out only under local anesthesia, with little or no antituberculous medication, using only primitive instruments and lighting.

Why is it that after several decades of infrequent use, thoracoscopic procedures are again gaining in importance throughout the world?

Jacobaeus himself believed that thoracoscopies could be used not only to divide adhesions but also to perform pleural biopsies, as an easy method for histopathological diagnosis of pleurisy. He was the first to describe endoscopic examination of pleural tumors. Unfortunately, early diagnosis of pleural malignancies today does not often lead to curative therapy. However, important palliation results from induction of a lasting pleurodesis performed by dusting talc during the thoracoscopy. Diagnosis of malignant mesotheliomas, and other pleural malignancies, may be made with facility at a relatively early stage, permitting therapeutic interventions which may prove more effective than those used in the past.

In addition to visualizing the pleural surfaces, the lung itself can be examined. In spontaneous pneumothorax, minute emphysematous bullous lesions and blebs, less than 1 mm in diameter, are seen in nearly all patients when examined with high-resolution equipment. It is therefore reasonable to assert now that there can be no "normal lung" in spontaneous pneumothorax. The information obtained via the thoracoscope in these patients is often superior to that seen by computer axial tomography (CT scan) or any other techniques short of thoracotomy.

The entire pulmonary mantle is accessible to the endoscopy examiner and his biopsy forceps, permitting diagnosis of peripheral pulmonary lesions, whether diffuse or localized, acute or chronic, benign or malignant. This technique makes it possible to perform certain tasks which were previously reserved for the surgeon: biopsy of the diaphragm, the pericardium, or mediastinal lymph nodes; sectioning of the sympathetic nervous system in vasculomotor syndromes of the upper limbs; clot lysis and hemostasis in hemothorax; disruption of loculations in empyemas; coagulation of blebs and bullae in spontaneous pneumothorax or of intrathoracic wounds by means of a YAG laser.

Thoracoscopy, while allowing full exploration of the thoracic cavity, is much less invasive and incapacitating than thoracotomy. Complications are uncommon and rarely occur when the procedure is performed by someone who has mastered the technique. The cost of treatment is much less than thoracotomy because of the shorter period of hospitalization, on average no more than 2–5 days. There are no sequelae as long as effective pleural drainage ensures complete pleurodesis. No rehabilitation is required and a normal active life can be resumed within a few days.

The use of thoracoscopy has been resumed partly as a result of considerable progress in modern techniques, particularly in the following two areas. (1) Endoscopic instruments have been greatly improved; telescopes now have an extremely high optical quality in spite of their very small diameter. (2) Progress in anesthetics allows for a wide choice that ranges from local anesthesia in outpatients to general anesthesia with endotracheal intubation. In practice, local anesthesia with neuroleptic sedatives has made thoracoscopy relatively simple and free of danger, allowing it to assume the role of standard treatment throughout Europe.

Lastly, techniques of the future are being evaluated. The use of biological adhesives in the treatment of spontaneous pneumothorax and chronic malignant effusions is a new possibility with thoracoscopy. The YAG and possibly other lasers, endoscopes with high magnification, microscopes designed specifically for endopleural examination, video microscopes, etc., all point the way to the future.

In view of the many possibilities of thoracoscopy, it is surprising that it is not performed even more often. There are several reasons for this. First, the technique of dividing adhesions in tuberculosis died out with the advent of effective antituberculous drugs in the early 1950s. During the same period the addition of percutaneous pleural needle biopsy (Cope 1958; Abrams 1958) to culture of pleural fluid aspirates confirmed the diagnosis in the vast majority of tuberculous pleurisy cases, thus replacing more invasive techniques. Thirdly, open surgical biopsy has become widespread as a result of the considerable progress made in thoracic surgical techniques with diminished associated morbidity. Thoracic surgeons in many medical centers, particularly in the English-speaking world, have often come to dominate pleural therapeutic procedures, as well as many diagnostic ones. This trend has gone so far that the simple placement of a chest tube, not generally complicated, has been reserved for the thoracic or general surgeon, even though the latter often has little expertise in thoracic diseases. On the other hand, pulmonologists in many centers leave thoracentesis and percutaneous pleural biopsy techniques to the youngest doctors in training, thus totally abdicating any role in manual techniques. With the number of chest specialists having increased exponentially in the last 15 years and the number of thoracic surgeons diminishing, pulmonologists need to regain control over the diagnosis and treatment of pleural diseases, just as the flexible fiberoptic bronchoscope, alveolar lavage, laser, etc. have permitted them to dominate the field of broncho-pulmonary diseases.

This practical manual therefore has two main goals. The first is to show that thoracoscopic techniques are simple, not overly invasive, require only a short stay in hospital (comparable with arthroscopic surgery), do not require expensive equipment and are within the capability not only of surgeons but also of any physician who is adept with his hands. The second is to emphasize the exciting aspects of this endoscopic procedure, with its wide variety of findings in the pleura, the diaphragm, the lung, and the mediastinum. Under direct vision a gross diagnosis is made within seconds, and confirmed by microscopy within hours, as in bronchoscopy and gastroenterologic endoscopy.

Therefore, any physician or surgeon who has an interest in the pleura should understand thoracoscopy. In diagnosing pleural effusions, thoracoscopy is only slightly more invasive than a simple percutaneous pleural needle biopsy but provides infinitely more information. In all cases where a chest tube is required, then it should take a pulmonologist only a few minutes to introduce first an endoscope via the same incision, if only to inspect the pleura and verify that the tube will be well positioned. Simplicity and effectiveness are thus the key words in modern thoracoscopy.

Chapter 1: History and Evolution of the Technique

Forlanini (1882), in Italy, described therapeutic pneumothorax, a procedure which facilitated closure of tuberculous cavities. In 1910, H.C. Jacobaeus in Stockholm published the first edition of his work "Concerning the possibility of using cystoscopy in the examination of serous cavities": he carried out laparoscopy and thoracoscopy, using the same type of equipment, with the aim of investigating the pleural cavity in cases of pleurisy. Later he reported 40 cases in which pleural adhesions were divided using his scopes (pneumonolysis) and in 1925, 120 cases included his thoracoscopic experiences in the diagnosis of pleural tumors (Jacobaeus 1925). Until the 1950s, however, thoracoscopy was almost exclusively used for pneumonolysis (also called "Jacobaeus' operation") throughout the world, whereas diagnostic thoracoscopy did not receive the recognition it merited; this was especially true in the United States and in the United Kingdom, where it was often considered as an invasive technique reserved only for surgeons (Lilienthal 1922; Alexander 1937).

Some teams, nevertheless, believed the technique should be developed as a means of diagnosis, and suggested extending it to the whole pleural pathology (Lelong and Meyer 1938; Sergent et al. 1939; Fourestier and Duret 1943; Sacco 1952; Lloyd 1953; Sattler 1961, 1966). Authors such as Touraine (1960, 1962, 1965) and Titscher and Hatzenberger (1974) emphasized the endoscopic appearance of malignant pleural disease and the contribution of biopsy under direct vision via the thoracoscope. At the same time, endoscopic studies of nontuberculous spontaneous pneumothorax were being carried out by Coulaud and Deschamps (1947).

During the 1960s there were several important studies: a large study by Brandt (1971–1978); Sattler (1981), whose first publication dates back to 1937; a large series by Bergquist and Nordenstam (1966); and Swierenga (1974, 1977) whose studies covered more than 1000 thoracoscopies, of which 317 were performed for pleural effusion. Since then, we have witnessed a veritable explosion of publications covering the experience of many authors in the diagnosis of tuberculous or malignant effusion and of spontaneous pneumothorax (books by Alcozer and Dorigoni 1984; Brandt, Loddenkemper et al. 1985; Quetglas et al. 1985; videofilm by Tassi and Marchetti 1988, etc.).

All of this experience was brought together at the first International Symposium on Thoracoscopy which we organized in Marseilles in May 1980. It was attended by participants from 16 countries (Boutin et al. 1981b, c, d). Another comprehensive symposium on thoracoscopy was organized in Berlin in 1987 (Loddenkemper 1989), which was on the current state of the art. Widespread interest in the technique has thus been established, and demand for the training of pulmonologists is high since our "Practical course on Thoracoscopy" that we have given in Marseilles since 1980 has attracted over 300 European physicians so far.

For a more complete history of the technique, one may refer to the reports of Le Tacon (1981) and Brandt et al. (1985). From the very beginning, rigid tubes were used. The Jacobaeus-Unverricht thoracoscope, manufactured by Wolf, using a 3-V electric bulb as its distal light source and with a 90° angle of view, was the most commonly used; two points of entry were necessary. Kremer's thoracoscope provided direct vision, while Kalk's had an oblique angle of view, combining the advantages of both lateral and direct viewing instruments (Wolf 1979). Guelbring's thoracoscope had very high optical quality with a wider field of view and excellent luminosity, but it was significantly larger in diameter (Douady and Meyer 1942). Twenty years ago Storz' thoracoscope still used the principle of a distal light source, which was then replaced by a quartz light guide, allowing endothoracic photography using flash. Films and photography could be carried out using Fourestier's universal endoscope (film by Gernez-Rieux and Voisin 1966) or Wolf's thoracoscope, developed by Brandt in Berlin.

A mediastinoscope can be used as a thoracoscope (Weissberg et al. 1981). Deslauriers (1976) performed mediastino-pleuroscopies under general anesthesia in 275 patients, starting with a conventional mediastinoscopy using Carlens' technique. Then, if a histopathological diagnosis could not be obtained, he digitally opened the mediastinal pleura and biopsied the visceral pleura. When necessary, the apex of the lung was pulled through the cutaneous incision and biopsied outside the body, followed by coagulation of the biopsy site. Lewis et al. (1976) also described a technique of direct access to the pleura using a mediastinoscope: with the patient lying on his healthy side, a cutaneous incision is made in the thoracic wall and the mediastinoscope is inserted. The effusion is then aspirated and air is insufflated. It is then possible to inspect the pleural cavity and suspicious areas are biopsied. Maassen (1972, 1975, 1981, 1989) described a similar technique which was also used by Nadjafi et al. (1976): in spite of pleural adhesions, a direct approach to the lesions allowed pleural or lung biopsies to be performed without difficulty. Maassen, like Deslauriers, also performed large pulmonary biopsies by extracting part of the lung through the cutaneous incision, and then coagulating or suturing the biopsy site as in a "wedge resection." The results of 173 cases were published by Werdermann et al. (1974). This technique, however, was closer to a minithoracotomy than a thoracoscopy and resembles surgical biopsy as described by Gaensler et al. (1964), since an endoscope was no longer necessary.

"Direct" thoracoscopy can be used on a patient whose visceral and parietal pleural surfaces are adherent. This method, inspired by Maassen's technique, involves making a cutaneous incision of about 2 cm over the lesion to be biopsied; after dissecting the intercostal space with blunt forceps, the parietal pleura is cleared with the finger as described by Light (1983), and the visceral pleura is freed using the index finger. In this way, a cavity is obtained which is large enough to perform biopsies using thoracoscopy forceps.

Alternatively, Ash and Manfredi (1974) and Boushy et al. (1978) used small arthroscopes, 10 cm in length and 1.7–2.2 mm in diameter, to perform thoracoscopies under local anesthesia. The authors used Travenol's Tru-Cut needles for pulmonary biopsies and Vim-Silverman, Cope, or Abrams needles for pleural biopsies, using a second point of entry for the needle. This method does not lend itself well for use in a cavity as large as the pleural space: current endoscopes, being 4 mm in diameter, are approaching the diameter of an arthroscope, but their length is 30 cm, allowing visualization of the entire thoracic cavity.

A flexible fiberoptic bronchoscope can be used to carry out thoracoscopy (Ben Isaac and Simmons 1975; Gunnels 1978; Senno et al. 1974, 1975): after making a skin incision, the intercostal muscles are dissected and the bronchoscope can be inserted either directly or inside a rubber chest tube or a metal sheath. The pleural fluid is aspirated through the suction channel and an equivalent amount of air is then insufflated. The induced pneumothorax allows inspection of the pleural cavity and biopsies to be carried out; afterwards, the pleural air is aspirated and the incision closed with a purse-string suture (Kerby et al. 1975). Although Gunnels indicates that this method might be very efficient, it should be noted that two of Kerby's patients and three of Senno's patients (1975) had to undergo thoracotomy after negative fiberoptic thoracoscopy. Oldenburg and Newhouse (1979) compared flexible thoracoscopy with thoracoscopy using a rigid instrument and concluded that the latter was the superior technique. Davidson et al. (1988) reached a similar conclusion.

It is therefore best to use rigid instruments designed specifically for use in the pleural cavity, i. e. thoracoscopes. Indeed, rigid thoracoscopes have a larger field of vision and allow larger biopsies to be taken. Rigid equipment optimizes use of diathermy coagulation and Nd:YAG laser, and still photography, films and video are far superior. Recently, manufacturers have produced rigid telescopes of diameters as small as 4 mm with exceptionally high quality lenses (Wolf's Panoview), much better than the optics of flexible fiberscopes.

Chapter 2: Equipment

As mentioned previously, a rigid thoracoscope with a cold light source is used in most cases. Its design must satisfy two requirements: (1) to make high-quality visual exploration and faultless photographic or video documentation, and (2) to facilitate multiple, large biopsies of sufficient size to ensure a definitive histopathologic diagnosis, while accomodating electrocautery and/or YAG laser cautery when necessary.

2.1 The Thoracoscope

We use equipment that we have developed in conjunction with the firm of Richard Wolf. These instruments, which have given us the best results are made up of several parts.

2.1.1 Trocars (Fig. 1)

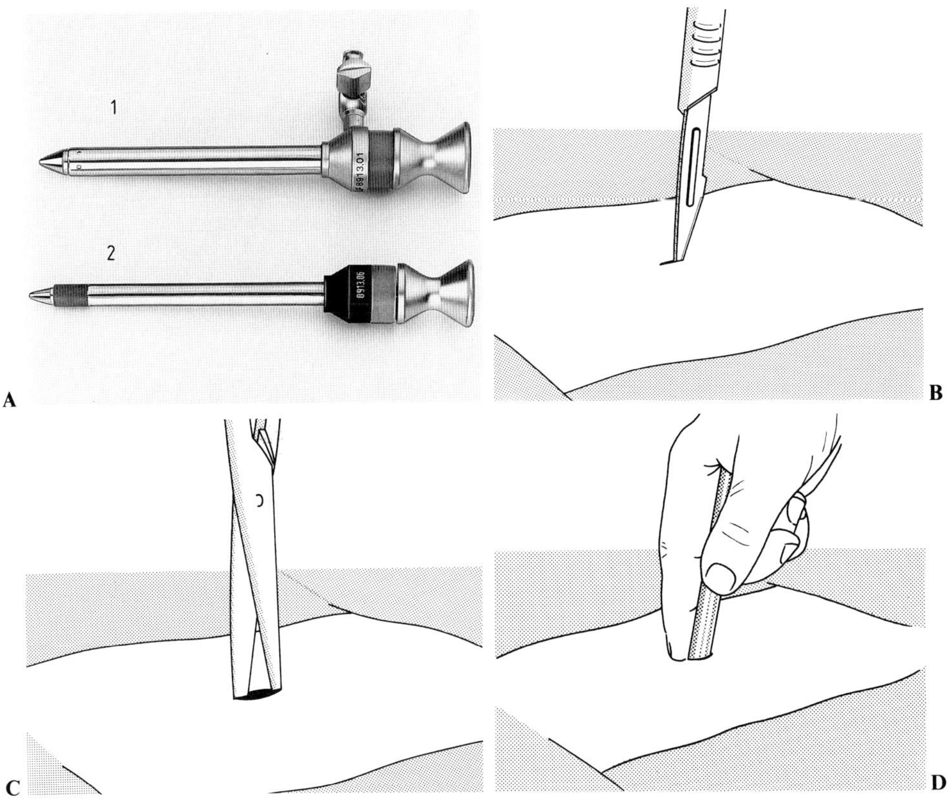

Fig. 1 A–D. Trocars. **A** *1:* 7-mm diameter trocar with a lateral tap. It is inserted gently under local anesthesia after a cutaneous incision has been made, and the intercostal space dissected using blunt forceps or straight scissors. *2:* 5-mm diameter trocar. Hardly any larger than Abrams needle. It is even possible to use 4 mm trocars with the new Panoview telescopes. **B** Incision. **C** Blunt dissection. **D** Inserting the trocar

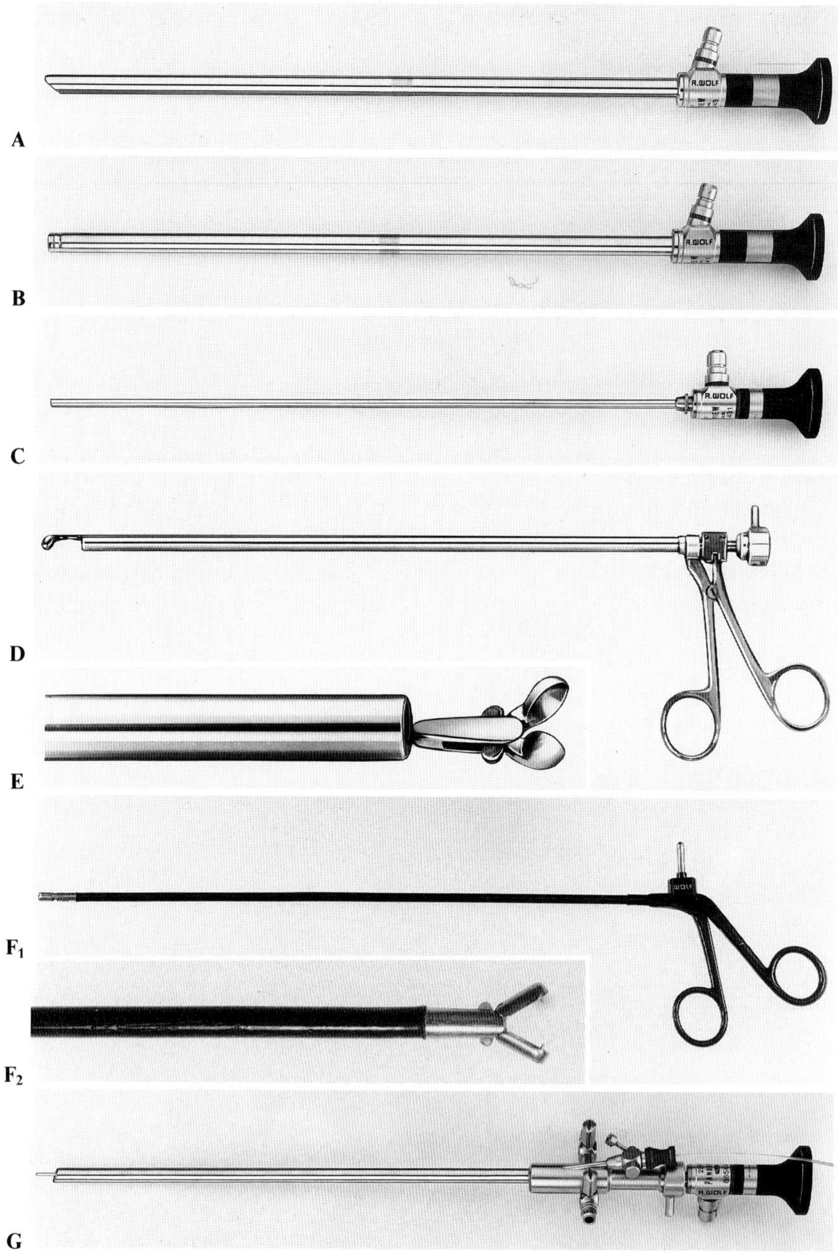

Fig. 2 A–G. Telescopes and forceps. **A** 7 mm Panoview with lateral viewing (50° oblique angle of view) for panoramic exploration of the entire pleural cavity. **B** Examination telescope, Panoview, 7 mm in diameter × 350 mm, for direct vision, (0° angle of view), allowing high quality exploration and easy video, film and photographic documentation. **C–E** Optical biopsy forceps for biopsies under direct vision with a single point of entry: **C** 4-mm direct vision telescope, **D** forceps, **E** close up view. **F** biopsy forceps: *1,* double spoon forceps connected to an electro-cautery for use with a 5 mm trocar via a second point of entry. *2,* Close up view. These three endoscopes and the forceps are all that is necessary to carry out a high quality exploration. **G** the laser thoracoscope, 7 mm in diameter for use with a single point of entry. The laser light guide can be inserted through a special channel visible on the bottom.

* All these materials are available from: Richard Wolf GmbH, Postfach 40, D-7134 Knittlingen

Trocars consist of an obturator and canulas, or sheaths. To make the examination easier, trocars should not be too large. We began our experience with trocars which were 12 mm in diameter and then changed to 10-mm trocars which were still difficult to manipulate in all directions when the intercostal space was narrow. Furthermore, the examination was sometimes limited by pain caused by the trocar pushing against the ribs.

The optimum diameter should therefore not exceed 5–7 mm. A lateral tap can be used at the beginning of thoracoscopy to aspirate fluid or insufflate air.

Our trocar of 7 mm in diameter and 100 mm in length is easy to insert. It is not airtight like a laparoscopy trocar, allowing air to enter and leave the cavity freely. The equipment can be made airtight when necessary, however, using a detachable rubber stopper.

Our 5 × 100 mm trocar is even easier to insert. The interior of the trocar is made of electrically insulated plastic, which avoids accidental burns to the chest wall while using electrocautery.

Even smaller trocars can accomodate the 4-mm Panoview telescopes, cytology brushes (Bejui-Thivolet et al. 1984), laser fiber, etc.

2.1.2 Telescopes

The optical quality of telescopes (Fig. 2) allows excellent visual exploration as well as good video, film, or photographic documentation. The new Panoview telescopes, which we are using extensively at this time, are perfect for our purposes. Panoview instruments with a 7-mm diameter are best for photography, while 4-mm telescopes are easier to insert using even the smallest trocars.

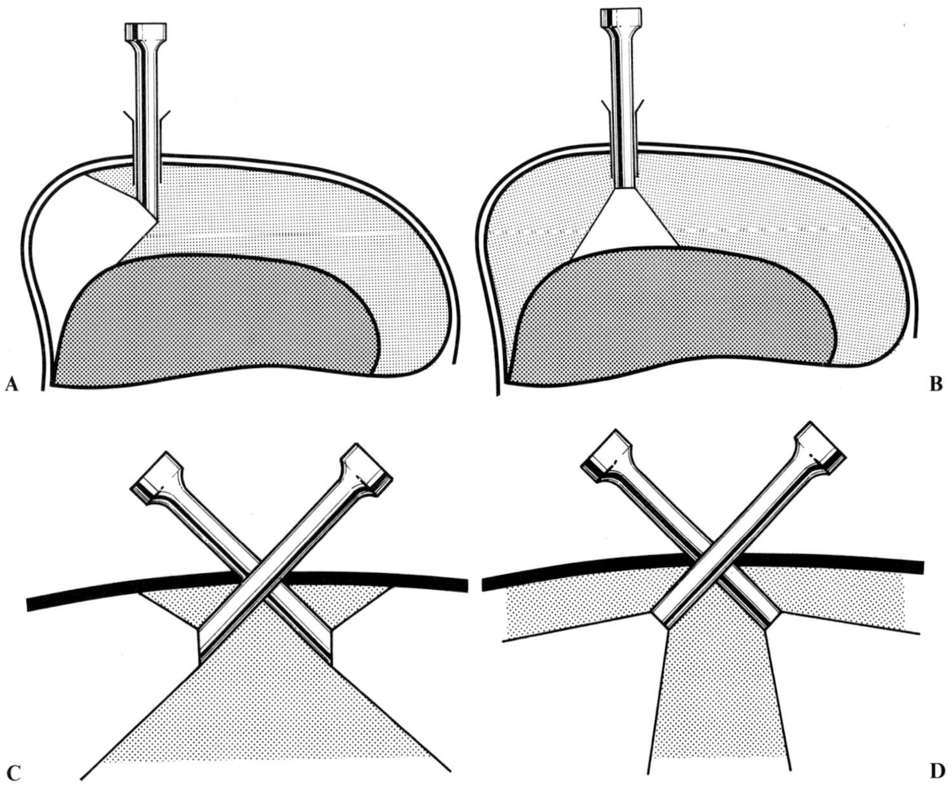

Fig. 3A–D. Exploration of the pleural cavity. A telescope with a 50° angle of view allows general, panoramic viewing of the cavity. Details can be seen in close-up using a telescope with a 0° angle of view, more adapted to video recording and photographs. The telescopes can be moved up to 45° from the upright direction of entry; beyond that, the pressure against the ribs becomes painful. **A, B** Using telescopes with 50° and 0° angles of view will virtually eliminate all blind spots during examination. **C** Vision through a telescope with 50° angle of view. **D** Vision through a telescope with 0° angle of view

Telescopes are available with various angles of vision, including 180° (straight ahead) and an oblique angle of view of 50°.

Telescopes with lateral or oblique angles of view are essential for an endoscopic examination since direct telescope does not allow looking back on the chest wall through which it has passed (Fig. 3). Although direct viewing may be more natural, one very quickly becomes accustomed to a lateral angle of view; by simply rotating the telescope, as a periscope, a superb panoramic view of the entire pleural cavity can be achieved. We therefore advise those who are learning the technique to use instruments with a 50° oblique angle of view from the beginning.

2.1.3 Forceps

The 7-mm optical forceps (Fig. 2) for biopsy under direct vision using a single point of entry is ideal for sampling the parietal pleura.

A 5-mm coagulation forceps is used for performing biopsies via a second point of entry through a 5-mm trocar. It is especially well suited for biopsying the diaphragmatic pleura, thick, hard, or fibrous pleural lesions, including asbestotic pleural plaques, and for sampling the visceral pleura and the lung.

2.2 Auxiliary Instruments and Accessories (Fig. 4)

1. Sheets, clamps, sterile gowns for the physician and his assistant
2. Needles, syringes, and cupula for the local anesthetic
3. Scalpels, compresses, suture, and anionic surfactant to prevent the formation of mist on lens surfaces (anti-fog solution, "Ultra-stop", Wolf)
4. Various forceps, needle holders, and clamps hemostats
5. Plastic aspiration tubes, 4 mm and 6 mm in diameter
6. Puncture needle for use under direct vision, 1.5 mm in diameter and 250 mm in length
7. Electrocautery loop for the lysis of adhesions
8. Swab
9. Talc atomizer (see Fig. 57)
10. Pleural drainage tubes (chest tubes), between 20 and 32 Fr
11. Guide for chest tube, or self-contained chest tube set with inner stylet
12. Light sources, cold light cables
13. Camera, video camera, color video tapes, and films, all of which can be sterilized under ultraviolet light
14. Endoscope warmer (see p. 22)
15. Manometer to measure pleural pressure (Figs. 5 and 7).

2.3 Endoscopic Photography

Two cameras were used to take the endoscopic photographs of this manual: (a) a Leica MDa, Visoflex 3, a 135-mm Elmar lens, f: 1/4, with an adaptor for a Wolf endoscope. This allows high quality photographs to be taken, which are, however, rounded on the four corners. (b) An Olympus OM2n with automatic winder was equipped with a Zuiko ×2 converter for doubling focal length, and a 85 to 120-mm Riwo zoom lens. It is therefore easy to enlarge up to four times on a 24 × 36 film, depending on the focal length used on the zoom lens.

Various reversible color films between 100 and 400 ASA for daylight photography were used, depending on the light absorption of the subject (which is stronger in reds), and were developed by means of a special procedure. Ektachrome 100 ASA is suitable for very "white" pleurae; Kodachrome 200 ASA was also often used. 400 ASA film was increased to 800 ASA when the subject was red or black.

The depth of field is limited to a few mm when taking full-frame close-up views.

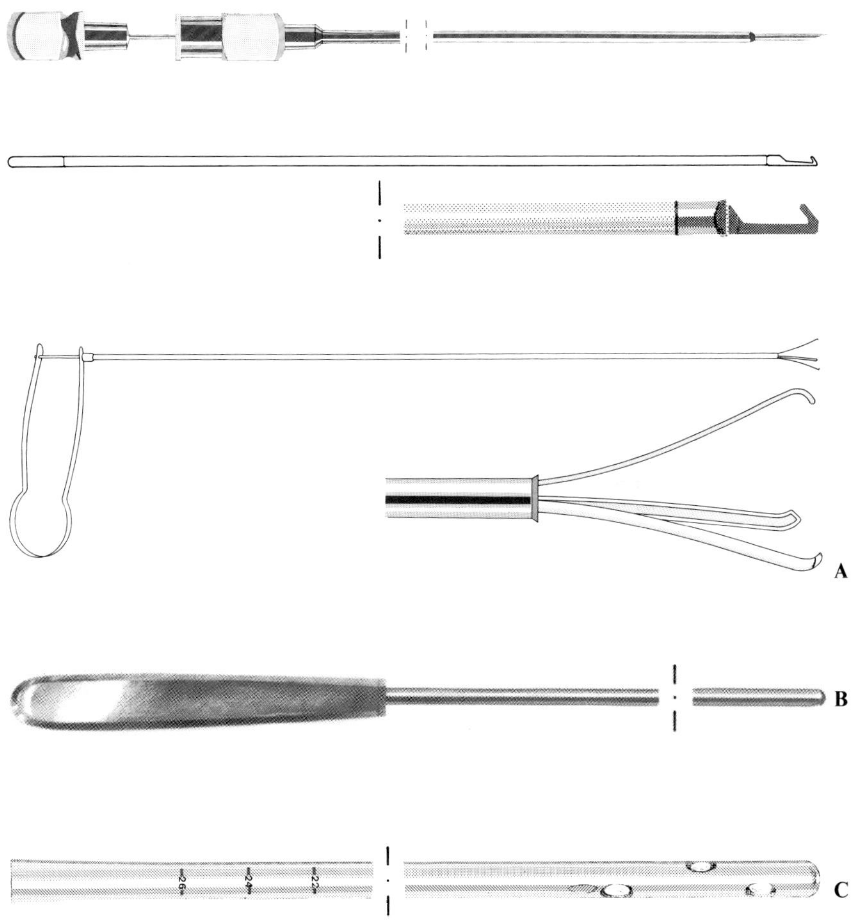

Fig. 4 A–C. Auxiliary instruments and accessories. **A** *Top to bottom:* a cytology puncture needle, 1.5 mm in diameter and 250 mm in length; an electrocautery loop to divide adhesions, 4 mm in diameter and 250 mm in length; grasping forceps with swab holder. **B** A blunt guide for inserting a drain, 5 mm in diameter and 500 mm in length; **C** a plastic 28 Fr drain, 500 mm in length

2.4 The Endoscopy Room

Thoracoscopies can be performed either in an operating room or in an endoscopy suite (Fig. 5). The room must contain the following:

1. A thoracoscopy table. This may be a simple operating table or, ideally, may have a height adjustment and a back which can be raised for operating in the semisitting position. Some tables can be adjusted laterally along a longitudinal axis which allows the patient to be repositioned easily (Brandt et al. 1985). Although these sophisticated tables are very useful, they are by no means essential.
2. Adjustable aspiration equipment for the pleural fluid, with 2-liter or more collecting bottles connected to negative pressure.
3. Simple anesthetic equipment, with air-feed and oxygen.
4. An overhead light with adjustable brightness.
5. A Mayo stand placed sideways across the surgical table to hold the instruments.
6. A 150-W HF scalpel for electrocautery, or an Nd:YAG laser.
7. Separate mobile carts for endoscopic light sources, photographic equipment, films, and videos.

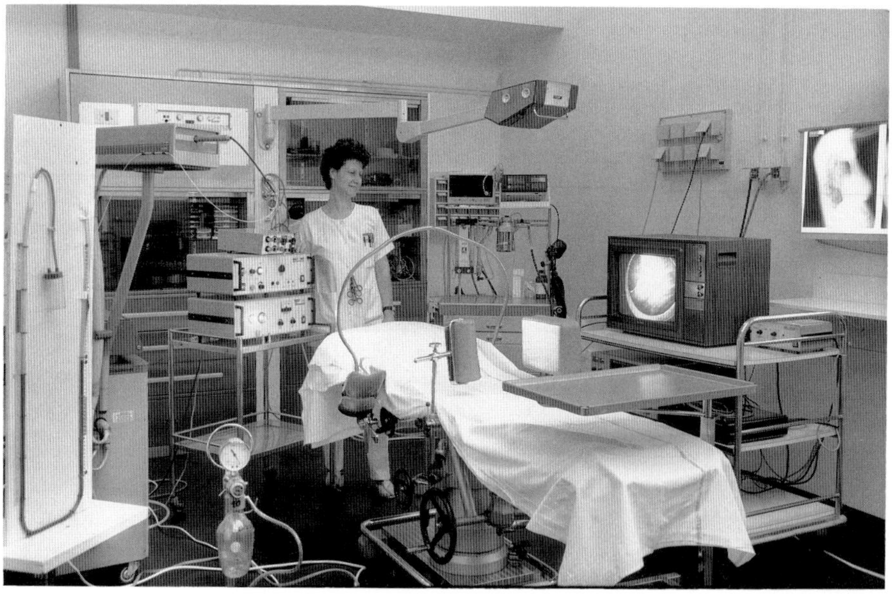

Fig. 5. The endoscopy room

8. A viewing box to display the patient's X-rays during the examination.
9. A stool.
10. A cupboard or drawers for different instruments.

2.5 Aseptic Conditions

Thoracoscopy must be carried out under sterile conditions. The room is sterilized in the same way as any other operating room. All the materials – the trocars, telescopes, forceps, all the accessories, the electrical connecting wires, the light-conducting fiberoptic cables, etc. – are sterilized after careful cleansing in trioxymethylene formalin. All cameras and equipment for photography, filming, and video recordings are sterilized using ultraviolet rays since formalin damages film. Talc is sterilized by autoclaving at 160° C.

The physician and assistant clean their hands with the standard surgical scrub technique and then put on sterile gown and gloves.

A remaining source of contamination is through the physician's eyes or eyebrows coming into contact with the telescope; one should therefore learn to look through the telescope without touching the eyepiece, the eye remaining a few centimeters away from the instrument. To avoid contact between the hand and the eye, the telescope should be held well away from the ocular, below the cold light connection.

The patient's skin is prepared by shaving and disinfecting a large area, so that different points of entry are possible, reaching from the sternum up to the clavicle, across the axilla past the scapula to the spinous processes and down as far as the base of the thorax.

Chapter 3: Thoracoscopy Technique

Although the present uses of thoracoscopy are fundamentally different from the original one, i. e. the lysis of adhesions, the actual technique of the operation itself has hardly changed. As before, an intimate knowledge of endopleural anatomy is essential, as well as is to skillfully manipulate the trocars, telescopes, forceps, and chest tubes.

3.1 Induced Pneumothorax

In order to insert the thoracoscope into the pleural cavity, pneumothorax must first be created. Examination is only possible if the pleural space between lung and chest wall is sufficiently large to move the instruments around easily and to visualize all important areas of the thoracic cavity. Ideally it should measure at least 10 cm on several X-ray views. To achieve this, most or all of the lung must be freed of the parietal pleural surface.

3.1.1 The Pleural Trocar (Fig. 6)

A pleural trocar for making punctures, measuring 2 or 3 mm in diameter and 100 mm in length, is ideal for inducing pneumothorax. Apart from the old trocars used to create therapeutic pneumothorax in tuberculosis (Kuss' trocar) no standard instrument is available. Ordinary needles commonly used for thoracentesis are very sharp and, therefore, involve a definite risk of lung puncture, particularly when the lung reexpands

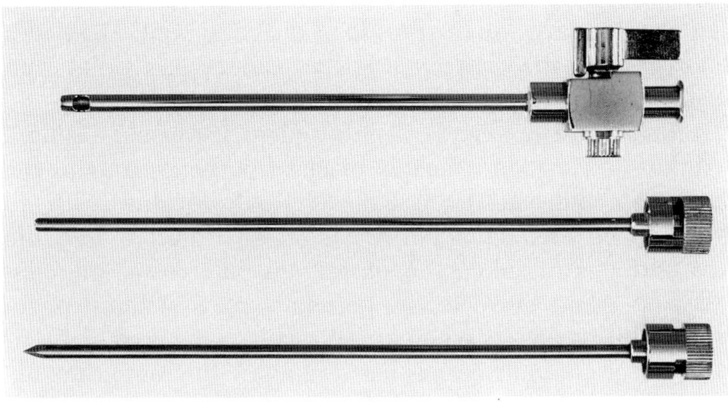

A

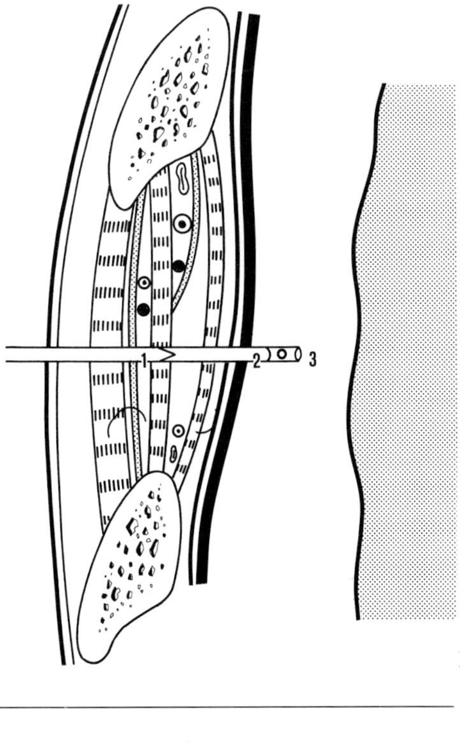

B

Fig. 6 A, B. The pleural trocar. **A** A pleural trocar, 2 or 3 mm in diameter, 100 mm in length (manufactured by Lepine, Lyon). From the *top:* trocar with tap, blunt obturator and, pointed obturator. **B** After local anesthesia. *1,* The skin and intercostal tissue are penetrated using the pointed obturator. *2,* The blunt obturator is used to pass through the parietal pleura. *3,* The trocar passes a few mm through the parietal pleura. It is blunt and does not traumatize the lung. Two openings on the tip of the trocar (a lateral and a distal one) ensure a complete evacuation of pleural fluid

during fluid removal. For this reason we use specially adapted instruments which are effective without this unnecessary risk. The trocar we have designed is available in two sizes: 2-mm diameter to aspirate simple effusions; 3-mm diameter for empyemas with thick fluid which is often difficult to aspirate through narrower bores.

The trocar contains a tap to control air exchange and a Luer connector for airtight connection of syringes and tubes. A pointed obturator allows passage through the skin and intercostal muscles without prior incision; a second blunt obturator is then inserted to pass safely through the parietal pleura without risk of puncture or laceration of the lung or diaphragm. This obturator also serves to clear the needle during puncture, should it become blocked with pus, fibrin, or blood. Tubes can be connected to the trocar so that any fluid can be aspirated or siphoned off. A side hole located distally on the trocar facilitates complete evacuation of the fluid.

3.1.2 On the Endoscopy Table

Pneumothorax may be induced a few minutes before thoracoscopy. Under local anesthesia, the pleural trocar is inserted and 200–300 ml of fluid at a time is aspirated through it, following which an equivalent amount of ambient air is allowed to enter by opening the trocar tap. The characteristic whistle of air can be heard as it passes through the trocar. Some physicians prefer to do this under fluoroscopic control (Brandt et al. 1985). As soon as the lung is in a state of equilibrium – an equal amount of air is heard entering the pleura during inhalation as leaving it during exhalation – the pleural trocar is removed and the thoracoscopy trocar is inserted. Aspiration of any remaining fluid is completed under direct vision through an aspiration channel fitted to the thoracoscope and connected to suction. It is very important that all fluid be aspirated before a systematic examination is begun, since any fluid left behind masks part of the pleural cavity and may obscure visual acuity through the thoracoscopic lens.

3.1.3 The Day Before the Examination

The patient is sometimes best studied when the procedure is performed the day before his scheduled thoracoscopy; this allows time to review his or her roentgenograms after the induced pneumothorax, in order to choose the best site of entry for the thoracoscope. Thus, posteroanterior, lateral, and oblique films – or biplane fluoroscopy – may indicate areas of pleural adhesions which are best avoided as a site of entry. Furthermore, pleural tumors that could not be appreciated on prior films are often evident after pneumothorax. This allows the practitioner to choose a site of entry rendering the biopsy a simpler task (Fig. 8).

The technique of pneumothorax differs depending on the absence or presence of pleural fluid.

(a) When there is no fluid. The puncture site is usually in the midaxillary area between the 3rd and 6th intercostal space, one or two fingerbreadths in front of the anterior edge of the latissimus dorsi muscle. Pleural adhesions in this area are rare. The patient lies on his healthy side with the head lowered, the arm raised over his head; a bolster or rolled-up sheet is placed on the table, under the patients's thorax. This position maximizes the spread of all intercostal spaces on the upside of the chest wall. The width of the intercostal spaces can be easily felt with the fingers through the skin and soft tissue.

The skin is disinfected in the usual fashion. Through a needle inserted perpendicular to the skin surface, 4–6 ml of 1% Xylocaine (with no added epinephrine) is slowly injected into the skin, subcutaneous fat, the intercostal muscles, and down to the parietal pleura, without penetrating it. When anesthesia is completed, a 2-mm pleural trocar is inserted along the same tract using the pointed obturator; this is exchanged for the blunt obturator when contact is made with the endothoracic fascia. The pleura provides resistance to further penetration, requiring a sudden, short, brisk jab of the blunt tool. A characteristic sound is heard as the parietal pleura is transgressed.

The blunt obturator is then removed, and the whistle of air entering the pleural cavity can be heard. At this point the manometer (Fig. 7) is connected using plastic tubing, and the pleural pressures are measured. The manometer will show large negative oscillations, usually ranging between −8 and −2 cm of water. The trocar tap is then reopened, and air is allowed to enter as the patient breathes in deeply three or four times. After some 300–500 ml of air has entered, pleural pressure is reassessed to document its continued negative value.

Straightforward cases, of course, are not difficult. In cases where there are adhesions in the area of entry, force should not be applied to the trocar and no attempt should be made to pass through tissue which offers unusual resistance. The manometer will register little or no movement if the pleura is not free. If the lung is accidentally pierced, the manometer will register low amplitude oscillations around the zero point. When it is impossible to achieve the pneumothorax from this area, the area further back, level with the latissimus dorsi muscle, may be tried; if this also fails, then the 2nd and 3rd intercostal spaces anteriorly should be attempted with the patient lying on his back. However, the number of attempts at entry during any one session must be limited for the sake of patient comfort.

To measure the quantity of air allowed to enter the thoracic cavity, one can use a pneumothorax apparatus or a similar setup (Brandt et al. 1985). In any case, the intrathoracic pressures must remain negative: insufflating air under positive pressure may induce mediastinal shifts, compromise cardiovascular performance, and could be painful to the patient.

Creating a pneumothorax is clearly more difficult when no effusion is present, but is quickly mastered with experience.

(b) When pleural fluid is present. The procedure is easier and has been described above in Sect. 3.1.2. When inducing pneumothorax the day before thoracoscopy, more ample time is allocated to pressure measurements and the presence of trapped lung is more likely to be anticipated (Light et al. 1980a); this can also reduce the actual time spent in a busy operating room. Although we have always replaced the fluid with ambient air, others have preferred to insufflate CO_2 as in laparoscopy (Brandt et al. 1985).

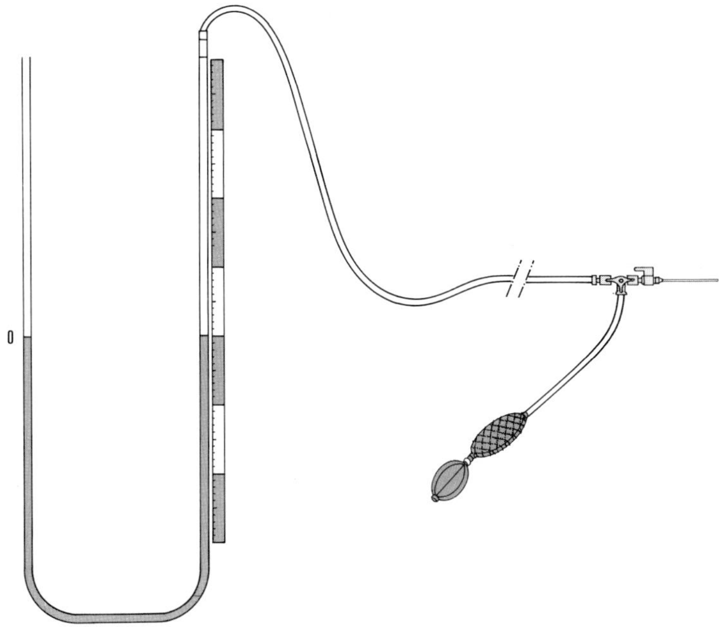

Fig. 7. Induced pneumothorax: measuring pleural pressures. From *right* to *left:* pleural trocar, three-way stopcock, rubber bulb to clear the liquid in the tubes during puncture, water manometer

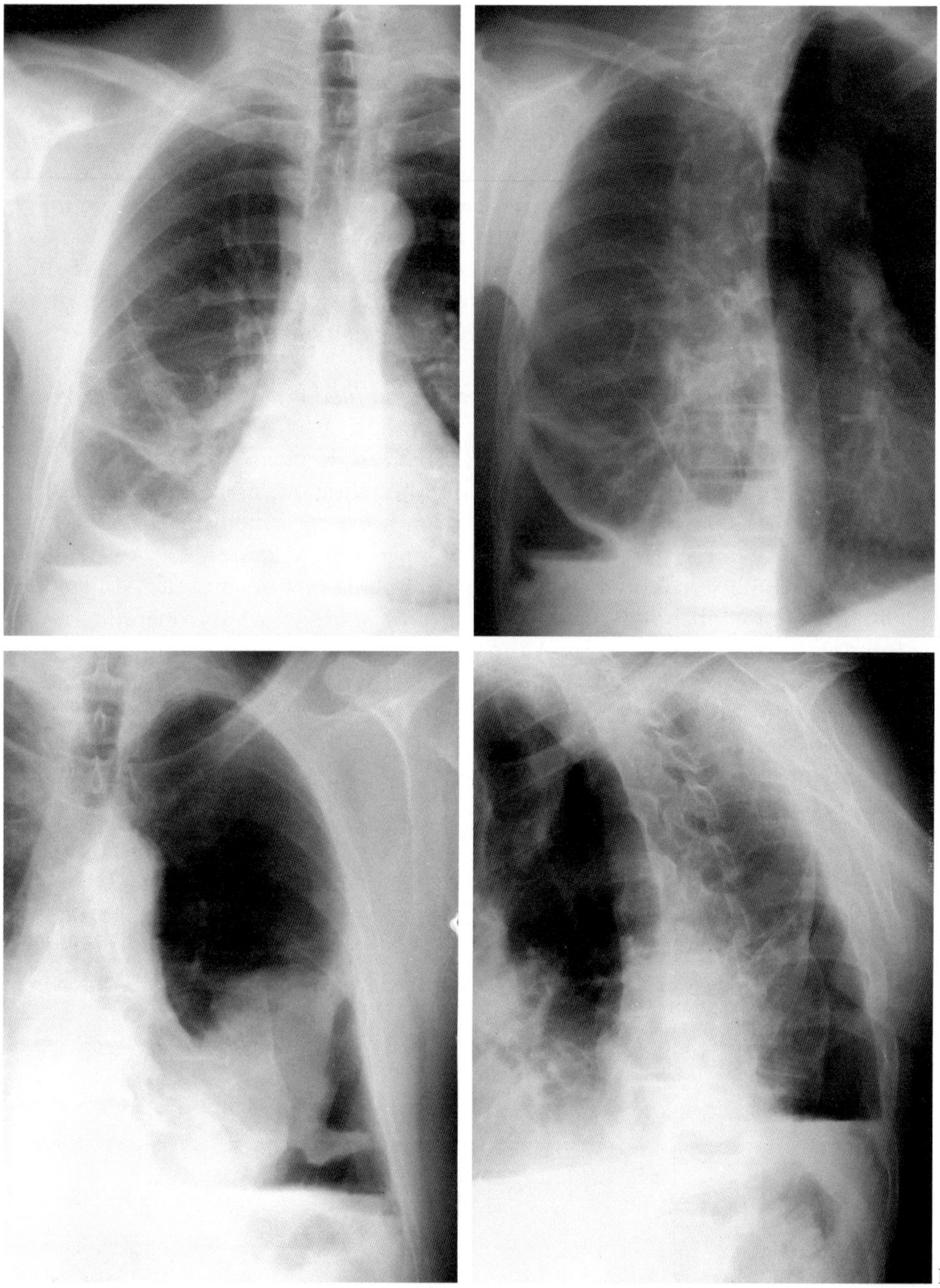

A B C D

Fig. 8 A–D. X-rays of induced pneumothorax. **A** Frontal X-ray: A hemorrhagic, loculated effusion is visible on the right. After evacuating 200 ml of fluid and injecting air, the pleural space is seen to be highly compartmentalized in this view. An air-fluid level above the diaphragm can also be noticed. **B** Right anterior oblique view: the superior level of the fluid is easily seen at the posterior axillary line, where the entry site will be located. The pneumothorax is more easily distinguished and appears larger than in the frontal view. **C** Frontal X-ray: a pleurisy with partitions is visible on the left side. **D** Left anterior oblique view: the induced pneumothorax appears larger than on the frontal view

3.2 Selecting the Point of Entry

3.2.1 The Standard Point of Entry (Fig. 9 A)

An axillary point of entry is selected in most cases. The axillary triangle has no large muscle obstructing passage of the instruments. It is bordered anteriorly by the lower edge of the pectoralis major muscle, posteriorly by the anterior edge of the latissimus dorsi muscle, and inferiorly at the level of the diaphragmatic insertions. Its apex reaches the second intercostal space. The point of entry is generally near the midaxillary line, within this triangle, and selected as follows: (a) in the 3rd or 4th intercostal space in patients with spontaneous pneumothorax, since the leak is usually in the upper lobe; (b) in the 5th, 6th, or 7th intercostal space for pleural effusions. The last two spaces are especially preferred when metastatic tumor and mesothelioma are suspected in order to reach the most common sites of these malignancies (Canto et al. 1977, 1981 a). This provides an excellent view of both the diaphragm and the costovertebral gutter. (c) in the 4th or 5th intercostal space for pulmonary biopsies so that all lobes can quickly and easily be reached.

While applying these principles carefully, we still sometimes find that certain key areas are not well seen or are inaccessible to the biopsy forceps, necessitating a second point of entry (see Sect. 3.9)

3.2.2 Point of Entry for Specific, Localized Lesions

In unusual cases, other points of entry are used, depending on the clinical setting or the roentgenograms. For instance, the 2nd or 3rd anterior intercostal spaces are chosen in cases of pneumothorax when anterior and superior emphysematous bullae or blebs are suspected.

One must bear in mind that a pleural lesion which is too close to the point of entry cannot be viewed or biopsied with a rigid thoracoscope. The lesion is approached most easily from the opposite side (Fig. 9 B). Therefore, one should choose (a) for posterior lesions, the anterior axillary line; (b) for anterior lesions, the posterior axillary line; (c) for lateral lesions, the mid-clavicular line.

Every effort is made to identify the precise level of the lesion on the roentgenograms so that the appropriate intercostal space can be used for the point of entry. Several important *anatomical landmarks* must be kept firmly in mind:

1. The anteromedial end of the 2nd intercostal space is located by palpating the angle formed by the manubrium and the body of the sternum: the ribs can then be counted from top to bottom.
2. In the axillary hollow, the 2nd intercostal space is the highest space that can be felt on a non-obese patient.

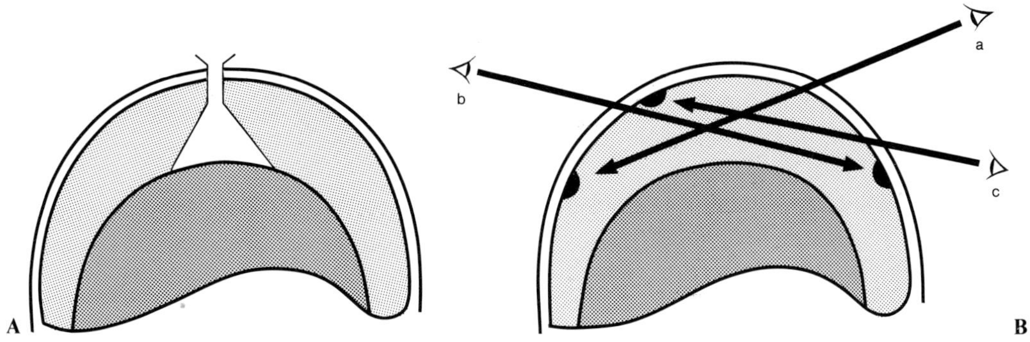

Fig. 9 A, B. Selecting the point of entry. A single point of entry is usually all that is necessary. However, creating a second point of entry being so easy, one should not disregard the extra advantages it affords in some cases (see Sect. 3.9). **A** The standard point of entry on the midaxillary line. *left*, posterior; *right*, anterior. **B** The position of the lesions to be biopsied determines the point of entry which should be on the opposite side, facing them: *a*, anterior axillary line to biopsy posterior lesion; *b*, midclavicular line for lateral lesion, *c*, posterior axillary line for anterior lesion

3. The ribs can also be numerated in the back, using the dorsal spinous processes. The reference point here is the prominent C7 spine, from which the vertebrae and ribs may easily be counted.
4. The ribs of a patient in the lateral position can be counted along the midaxillary line: the lowest rib which can be felt is the tenth; the 11th and 12th floating ribs are behind. The ribs can then be counted from the bottom upwards.
5. The male nipple is generally situated near the level of the fourth rib.
6. If an anterior point of entry is selected, remember that the internal mammary artery and vein pass just posterior to the ribs some 16 to 18 mm lateral to the sternal margin.
7. When erect, the liver is very high within the thorax, reaching as far as the fourth intercostal space during forced exhalation. However, in the left lateral decubitus position, gravity pulls the liver away from the chest wall and there is little possibility of injuring it. Avoiding the liver should be a simple matter once the insertion levels of the diaphragm and the dimensions of the costophrenic angle are appreciated radiographically. Lateral decubitus films or fluoroscopy provide an extra margin of safety when a low entry site is planned. In the event that confusion of landmarks or insufficient caution results in the trocar meeting the liver, significant hepatic capsular injury can usually be avoided by withdrawing at the very moment the practitioner feels the change in resistance to penetration.
8. Although radiographic review is mandatory in each patient, one should keep typical diaphragmatic anatomy in mind: the diaphragm is more or less symmetrical on both sides; it starts anteriorly just below the sixth costal cartilage at about the same height as the xiphoid process, slopes downwards towards the side, and reaches its lowest point level with the end of the eleventh rib and the second lumbar vertebra, approximately in the mid-axillary line. Then it rises again towards the back, crossing the 12th rib 8–9 cm from the spine and joins the upper edge of the first lumbar vertebra (Fig. 10).
9. Remember that the major fissure crosses the mid-axillary line at the fourth intercostal space on the right – the minor fissure begins at this point – and at the 5th intercostal space on the left.

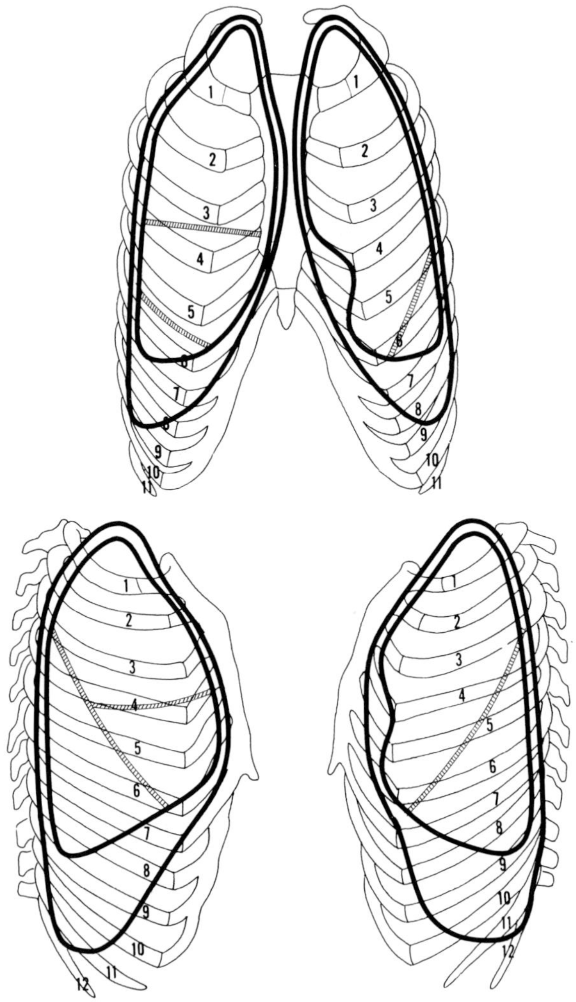

Fig. 10. Anatomy of the pleura as related to the chest wall, the diaphragm and fissures. The diaphragm reaches its lowest point level with the end of the eleventh rib. Its situation is more or less symmetrical on both sides. The fissures: remember that a chest tube inserted in the mid axillary zone, in the 4th intercostal space on the right or the 5th intercostal space on the left, may directly penetrate the fissure and become ineffective

3.3 Anesthesia

3.3.1 Premedication

The fasting patient is given intramuscular premedication 1 h before examination. According to local custom, a wide variety of agents may be administered, including 50-100 mg of pethidine or demerol, 5-10 mg of diazepam, 25-100 mg of hydroxyzine, etc. Atropine, 0.25 mg or more, may also be given to minimize chances of vagal reactions.

3.3.2 Local Anesthesia

Many authors prefer local anesthesia (Bergqvist and Nordenstam 1966; Fleishman et al. 1956; Guérin et al. 1989b; Loddenkemper 1981; Vanderschueren 1981b; Rusch and Mountain 1987, etc.) which has the advantage of being quick and simple, putting little stress on the patient. There are practically no contraindications except in patients allergic to the anesthetic and those with a hemorrhagic diathesis. It does, however, require a confidence-inspiring, well-trained, skillful physician who is able to avoid causing pain and discomfort to the patient.

Local anesthesia is always advisable if the thoracoscopy can be performed quickly in a pleural cavity free of adhesions and if no complications are foreseen. It is also preferred over general anesthesia in high-risk patients with poor general health, limited respiratory function, or cardiac decompensation.

Method: a syringe with 10-20 ml of Lidocaine 1% (or Bipuvacaine) with 1/100000 adrenalin is attached to a small-bore needle for intradermal injection, followed in turn by subcutaneous and intercostal muscle infiltration down to the parietal pleura. Following a path perpendicular to the skin surface ensures that the entire straight path of the instruments will be pain-free. Entry into the pleural cavity is confirmed by drawing back on the syringe, which is seen to fill with air or fluid. Adrenalin is used to minimize the chances of blood oozing from the internal side of the entry point: indeed, even a few drops of blood may course along the trocar distally and obscure the thoracoscope lens each time it is inserted. When this happens, the scope must be frequently removed for cleansing, which unnecessarily delays the procedure.

3.3.3 "Neuroleptanalgesics"

Modern drugs which combine properties of sedation, analgesia, and amnesia are excellent adjunctive medications. Sedative qualities help allay anxiety, which is present to variable degrees in nearly every patient. Analgesia reduces the discomfort some patients experience during parietal pleural biopsy, or when the lung is reexpanded to the chest wall after talc insufflation. As for amnesia, it is widely felt to be of importance by anesthesiologists today. Dosing may be kept flexible according to the physician's wishes and the needs of the patient, insuring an early discharge of the patient from the operating room. Popular neuroleptanalgesics include 5-10 mg Droperidol, or 40 mg Nefopam or 5-10 mg Pethidine, 5-10 mg Midazolam or 5-10 mg Diazepam, and 50 mcg Fentanyl.

3.3.4 General Anesthesia

General anesthesia may be administered by mask with spontaneous ventilation. On the other hand, the patient may be intubated, permitting ventilation to be assisted or controlled by the anesthesiologist.

In the past, we and many others (Boutin et al. 1979; Bloomberg 1970, 1978; Canto et al. 1985a, 1989; Pepper 1978; Rodgers and Talbert 1976; Rodgers 1979, 1979a), often elected to use general anesthesia with endotracheal intubation. That permitted us to perform unlimited biopsies and to section widespread adhesions without fear of patient discomfort. Painless electrocautery could be performed, and we had time to take some high quality photographs and films during the procedure, without feeling rushed. It was and still is the preferable technique when selective intubation simplifies work best performed on an immobilized lung, as for laser work in general and for cauterizing pleural blebs in spontaneous pneumothorax.

3.3.5 Conclusion

As a practical matter today, we prefer the lightest anesthesia possible, usually a simple combination of premedication, local anesthesia and a neuroleptic, which permits the patient to remain conscious as much as reasonably possible during the procedure and does not preclude prompt awakening as soon as the lung is reexpanded to the chest wall. One should not, therefore, give in to the unexperienced anesthetist who desires the security of intubation with its attendant risks of secondary respiratory depression. Nowadays, endotracheal intubation should be elected only when the practitioner determines that the procedure requires it.

3.4 Position of the Patient

3.4.1 Lateral Decubitus (Fig. 11)

When a standard point of entry has been chosen, the patient usually lies in lateral decubitus position, with the healthy side down. He must be in a comfortable position, especially if the examination is performed under local anesthesia. Patient movements during the procedure may be minimized with the help of straps, adhesive tape, or cushioned supports attached to the table. The head rests on a pillow. A round bolster is slipped under the thorax to arch the vertebral column convexly upward, thus enlarging the intercostal spaces. This makes it easier to position and maneuver the trocar in any direction. The upper arm is raised at a right angle which further widens the intercostal spaces. The forearm is strapped to a supple metal cradle with gauze bandages, or held up in a sling. The arm can also be left in a high horizontal position with the forearm flexed over the head. The patient is grounded by placing a metal plate between the table and one buttock.

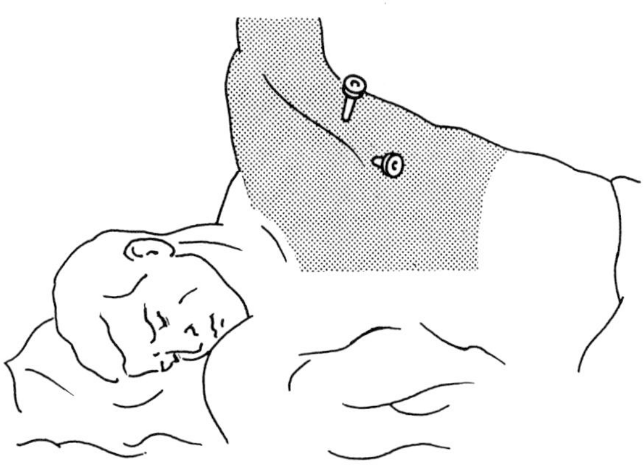

Fig. 11. The patient on the endoscopy table. The patient usually lies on his healthy side. Modern thoracoscopy methods are similar to older techniques. This illustration dates back to 1942 (Douady and Meyer). The position of the trocars may be different, however, since exploration now covers the entire pleural cavity, not just the apex, which was the primary interest of phthisiologists. In case of pleurisy, for example, points of entry are lower, around the 5th to 7th intercostal space. In spontaneous pneumothorax, a higher point of entry will be chosen, in the 3rd or 4th intercostal space

The physician usually faces the patient, while his assistant is across the table, behind the patient's back. The anesthetist or a second assistant stands at the patient's head to check the pulse, arterial blood pressure, respiration, and general well-being. A saline intravenous infusion is dripped slowly, to provide immediate access for any necessary medication. Oxygen is at hand. Continuous finger-pulse oximetry is reassuring, when available, for patients with severe respiratory problems – though in most patients hypoxemia does not significantly worsen during the procedure.

Brandt et al. (1985) use a table which can adjustably rotate the patient along both a longitudinal and an anteroposterior axis. This system uses gravity to move the lung into optimal positions: a Trendelenburg position is used to obtain a better view of the diaphragm; a semisitting position lowers the apex; and lateral rotation allows a more complete examination of the anterior and posterior portions of the pleura.

3.4.2 Dorsal Decubitus

The dorsal decubitus position is less complicated to set up and more confortable for the patient than lateral decubitus. It is used for three main entry points:

1. *An anterior point,* in the second or third intercostal space, allows exploration of the pulmonary apex and the pleural dome. This is

particularly useful in cases of spontaneous pneumothorax where anterior and superior emphysematous bullae and blebs are suspected. The superior portion of the dorsal sympathetic trunk can also be reached with this access (Guérin 1989, 1989a);

2. *A lateral point,* on the anterior axillary line in the third intercostal space, discloses the superior mediastinum with its superior vena cava and the brachiocephalic artery, the superior, anterior, and mid-mediastinal lymph nodes, and the azygous vein.
3. *A last point,* located on the anterior axillary line in the fifth or sixth intercostal space gives a good view of the pericardium. Note that biopsy of the pericardium is possible on the left side but is absolutely unwise on the right side, since the wall of the right atrium is quite thin and often adherent to the pericardium.

3.4.3 Ventral Decubitus

The ventral decubitus position provides access through the midaxillary line to the costovertebral gutter, as the lung falls to the front of the pleural cavity. It is rarely used and, indeed, is not very convenient for the practitioner.

3.5 Thoracoscopy Using a Single Point of Entry

3.5.1 Insertion of the 7-mm Trocar (Fig. 1)

After preparing the sterile field and administering local anesthetic, an 8- to 10-mm skin incision parallel with and in the middle of the selected intercostal space is made with a simple scalpel. Blunt dissection is then performed with straight scissors as far as the parietal pleura, in preparation for the trocar insertion. The trocar is pushed through this opening with moderate pressure; a sudden release of resistance is felt as the parietal pleura is penetrated, and the sound of air can be heard entering and leaving the thoracic cavity freely once the obturator has been removed.

Once the skin incision has been made, the trocar can also be inserted directly into the pleural cavity. In this case, the trocar should be held firmly in the palm of the hand and pushed downward, exactly perpendicular to the chest wall, with enough force to pass through the intercostal muscles and the parietal pleura. If the trocar is not skillfully handled, it might pierce the lung; this risk is greatest when the lung is close to the chest wall. The measured distance from chest wall to lung surface, based on the roentgenograms performed just after pneumothorax is induced, must therefore be kept firmly in mind.

Any fluid remaining in the pleura is aspirated using a blunt flexible plastic tube, which is fed through the trocar sleeve to the dependent areas of the thoracic cavity. The diameter of the tube should not be more than 5 mm so that there is still space between the walls of the tube and the trocar sleeve for air to enter the pleural cavity and replace the fluid being aspirated. In patients with large effusions, a sudden cough might flood the operative field; to avoid this, the lateral tap on the sleeve can be used to rapidly aspirate the effusion.

The same tap is also used to insufflate air when the lung does not spontaneously fall away from the chest wall.

Once the sleeve is in place, the assistant is responsible for keeping it in position, maintaining its end about 1–3 cm into the pleural cavity. Should the patient cough, the assistant immediately withdraws the sleeve until it is flush with the internal chest wall, in order to minimize risks of trauma to the lung.

3.5.2 The Thoracoscopy

As complete an examination as possible is made of the parietal and visceral pleura; only the posterior section and the mediastinal side of the lung cannot be seen. Using a 50° Panoview telescope, a circular panoramic view of the entire cavity can be achieved simply by rotating the endoscope (Fig. 3) without altering its direction or its depth. Depending on the patient's position, most of the superior and inferior mediastinum can be seen; the diaphragm, most lung surfaces, fissures, and pleural dome are all visible. With practice, the endoscope can be manipulated in all directions without pushing against the ribs; this is particularly important as it might otherwise be painful to the patient under local anesthesia.

Serous fluid sometimes obscures vision during the examination. The lens can be cleaned with anti-fog preparations such as Lauryl-sodium sulfate solution or "Ultra-stop" (Richard Wolf). A telescope warmer provides even further convenience as it prevents vapor from condensing on the lens: as soon as a telescope is changed, it is immediately placed in the warmer in order to be kept at a temperature of about 50° C.

There are often fine adhesions resembling a spider web (Fig. 15) which can hinder examination. These can easily be severed using a blunt probe or forceps, by insufflating air to further collapse the lung, or by cutting them with electrocautery.

3.6 Endoscopic Anatomy

Visual exploration is carried out in a few minutes by alternatively using the direct and the 50° telescopes. A probe enables the physician to push aside any fibrinous strands interfering with a clear view. There are always two levels of observation using telescopes: from a distance of 5–10 cm to obtain a wide-angle view with weak magnification; and then a close magnified view at a distance of 1–2 cm to inspect the cavity very carefully and to select the best biopsy sites.

3.6.1 The Pleura

In its normal state, the pleura is transparent (Fig. 12), allowing visualization of many structures through it, including the ribs, the parietal vascular pattern, the diaphragmatic insertions and central tendon, the pericardium with its attendant fat, the fibrous or fatty tissues of the pleural dome, the sympathetic trunk, the intercostal vessels, etc. Variable amounts of anthracotic pigment can occasionally be seen within the parietal pleura, especially posteriorly and in the costovertebral gutter (Fig. 13). These are often linear or canalicular, corresponding to the underlying lymphatics, or they may be punctiform like the lymphatic formations described by Kampmeier (1928).

Fatty collections are often abundant in the pleura, especially in obese people (Fig. 14). These may take the form of long yellowish or brownish plaques located along the ribs, in the apex, in the anterior mediastinum around the pericardium, and on the diaphragm.

Abnormal pleura. One of the hardest tasks for the endoscopist is to distinguish between innocuous and malignant or tuberculous "inflammation". In fact, it is often impossible to tell the difference just by looking, since in 13.5% of our cases (Table II; Boutin 1982b) invasive cancer has the appearance of simple inflammation.

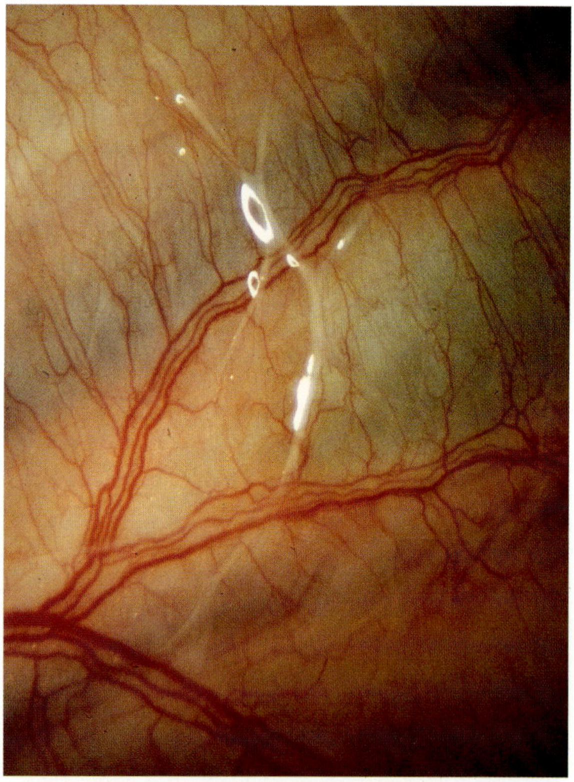

Fig. 12. A normal intercostal space. Under normal conditions, the pleura is transparent. The outline of the ribs is visible as well as the intercostal vessels, with their network of small arteries and venules. The pleura has usually a bluish white colour. Fine lymphatic vessels are sometimes visible in the form of whitish filaments

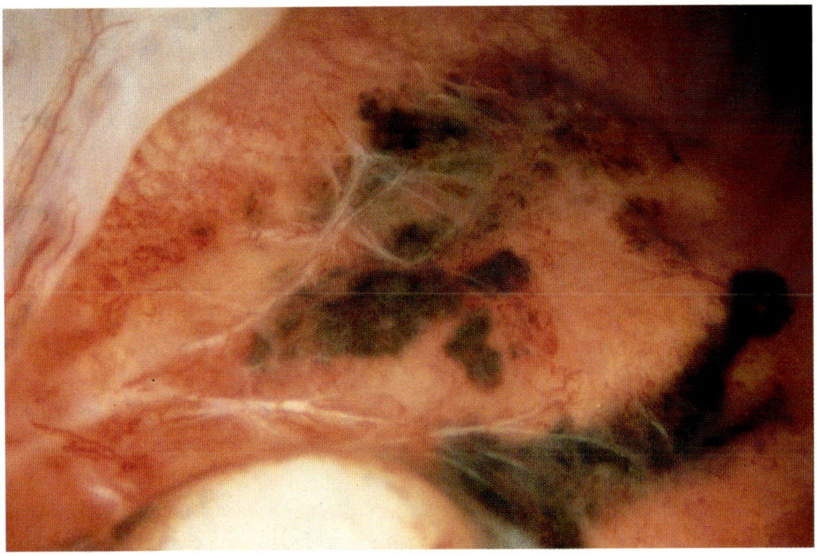

Fig. 13. Anthracotic pigment deposits, lymphatic vessels and malignant nodules on the parietal pleura. There are often bluish or blackish anthracotic deposits on the parietal pleura, especially posteriorly and inferiorly in the costovertebral gutter; they are either punctiform or linear, corresponding to lymphatic tissues affected by the pigment. Malignant nodules (at the *top* and *bottom* on the *left)* often develop in this area, suggesting an invasion via the lymphatic system: whitish threadlike lymphatic vessels close to the malignant nodules are about 0.1 mm in diameter

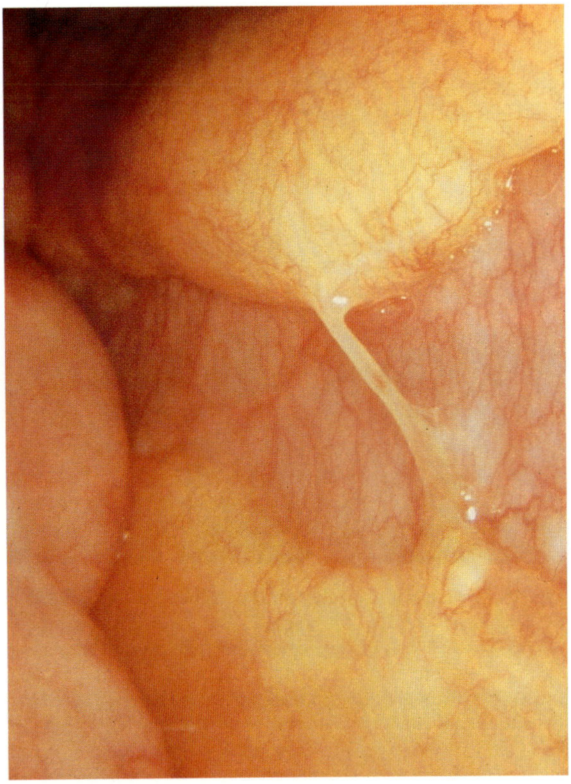

Fig. 14. Pleural fat. There are consistent amounts of fatty tissue in the pleural cavity, especially in overweight patients. It takes the form of yellowish or brownish masses in the apex, the mediastinum, around the pericardium and in the costodiaphragmatic gutter. Here, it forms large plaques along the internal side of the ribs and, in some places, along the intercostal space where the vascularity is easily visible. The normal lung is shown on the *left*

Simple inflammation is usually redder with a smoother, more regular surface and is more edematous than malignant pachypleuritis. When biopsies are taken, the forceps will cut a clear section of malignant tissue, whereas it easily pulls away much larger sections of inflamed pleura. However, this difference is only a matter of degree, and many biopsies should be taken (up to 15 or 20) in order to be certain that the pathologist has representative samples of the lesions which have been observed.

Nonspecific pleural inflammation (Figs. 15, 16) can be found in different stages:

- *Mild.* a simple increase in normal pleural vascularity, giving the pleura a pinkish hue; it is still thin and transparent.

- *Intense.* the pleura is bright red with engorged blood vessels and subpleural edema. The serosa becomes opaque and the outline of the ribs, arteries, and intercostal veins can no longer be distinguished. The pleura can be up to 3-5 mm thick. These changes are often more prominent in the costovertebral gutter and on the diaphragm; as the pleura is viewed upwards, frequently the pleura thins out, has progressively less reddish coloration, and finally may look completely normal at the apex.

- *Chronic.* In long-established pleurisies, the pleura remains as thick, but has a white or grayish tinge; it is opaque as a result of invasion by fibroelastic and collagenous tissue.

Specific pleural lesions. The following three patterns can easily be distinguished on a background of nonspecific inflammation: (a) lymphangitis appears as a fine reticular pattern covering all or part of the pleura (Fig. 17); (b) tuberculous or sarcoid granulomata are 1-3 mm in diameter. In sarcoidosis, they are much more common on the parietal pleura than is generally appreciated (see Fig. 54 and p. 62); (c) malignant nodules, which are variable in size and shape, usually predominate inferiorly (see Fig. 46 and 37).

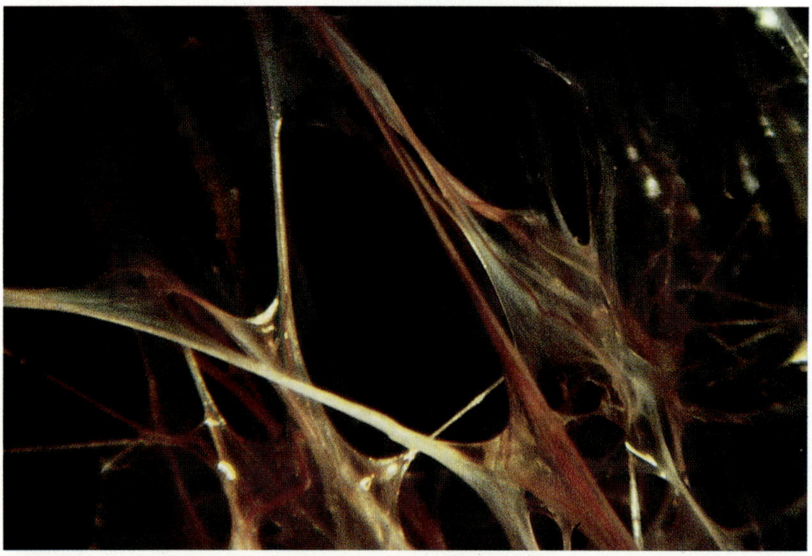

Fig. 15. Nonspecific inflammation. Adhesions are found in several forms: on this photograph, they are fibrinous, slack, avascular, and completely cover the bottom of the pleural cavity. They can easily be divided using forceps by proceeding slowly through what appears to be an impenetrable mass of adhesions, until the parietal pleura is reached. One can have difficulty recognising anatomical landmarks in a pleural cavity which is completely red and has several adhesions running through it, causing partitioning. If this happens, one should proceed as follows: *(a)* locate the diaphragm inferiorly: it moves as the patient breathes; *(b)* identify the lung in the center: it is soft when touched with the forceps; *(c)* identify the ribs on the external edge of the cavity: they feel hard to the touch. It is from this area that parietal pleural biopsies may most safely be taken

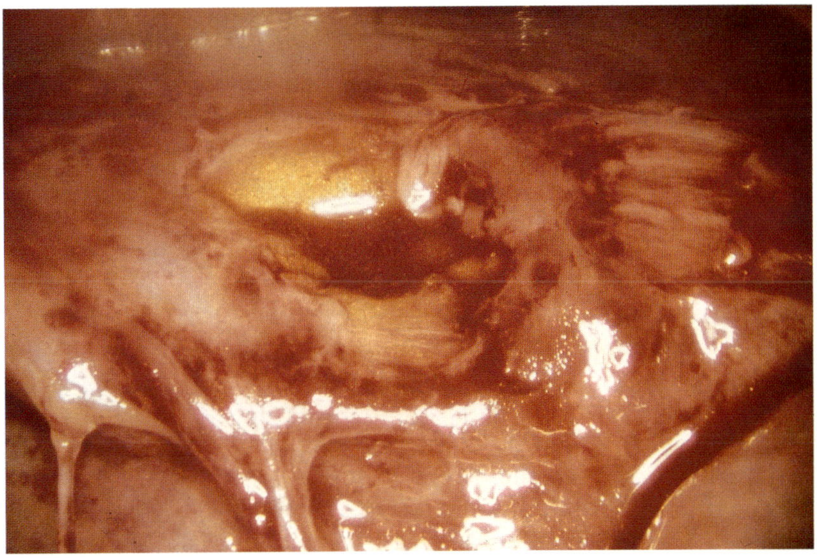

Fig. 16. Inflammatory pachypleuritis. This is another example of innocuous pleural inflammation. The pleura is thick, bright red and hemorrhagic. The fluid is clear. The thickness of the pleura can easily be inferred from the depth of the biopsy site in the *center* of the picture. Linear clusters of fibrin can be seen at the *bottom* of the photograph

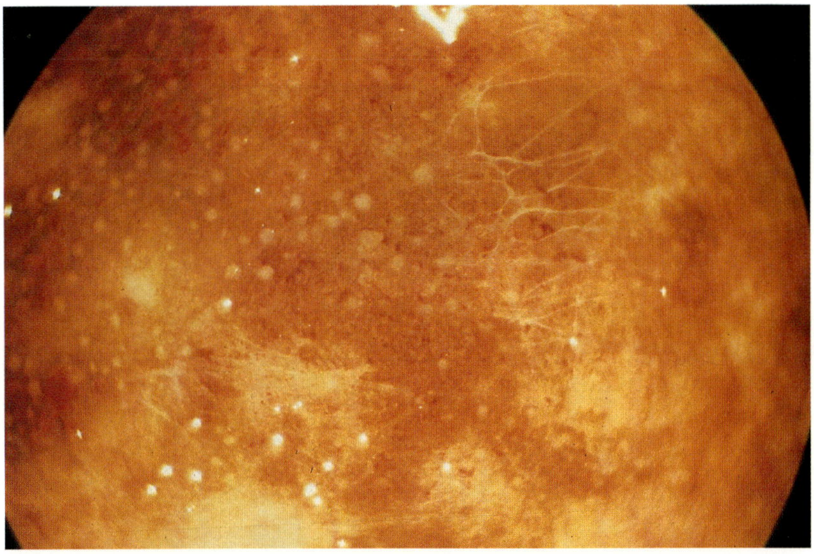

Fig. 17. Pleural lymphangitis in a chylothorax. The parietal pleura is completely covered with a network of lymphangitis. Nodules can be seen where the vessels join together. This photograph was taken from a distance of 5–6 cm using a wide-angle lens. It can be compared with Fig. 39 and 44 which were taken close-up with a telephoto lens: they show the advantage of taking pictures under high magnification revealing details which cannot be seen using normal or wide-angle lenses

3.6.2 **The Lung** (Fig. 18)

As seen through the 50° telescope, the lung looks like a cone, narrowing at the apex, sometimes with adhesions of variable importance between the visceral and parietal pleura. The fissures can easily be recognized (Fig. 19). Under normal conditions the surface is pink, soft and slightly shiny with a regular reticular pattern demarcating the pulmonary lobules. Black or blue star-shaped spots of anthracotic pigment are scattered over the surface.

The visceral pleura is normally transparent. When inflamed, it quickly becomes thick and pink, red, or white in color. Areas of atelectasis are purplish red, with clear edges (Fig. 20). Visceral lymphangitis, granulomas of miliary tuberculosis, and malignant nodules are quite visible and easy to biopsy. Umbilication of the lung surface is often seen with peripheral, subpleural malignancies. Probing with forceps reveals a hardened surface which resists deformation.

In cases of pulmonary fibrosis, the lung surface takes on an irregular shape, with numerous small emphysematous bullae protruding from the surface.

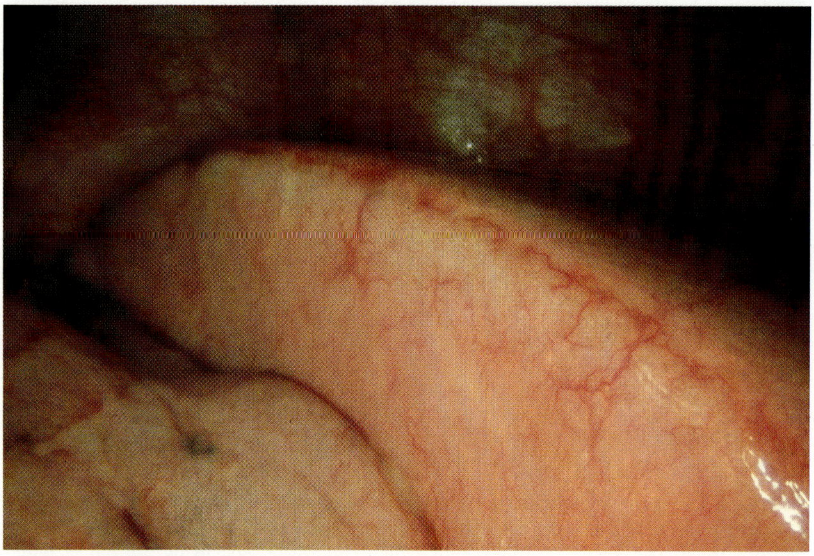

Fig. 18. Normal lung surface. Under normal conditions the lung is pink. This is a left lung with the upper lobe on the *right* and the lower lobe on the *left*. The fissures can easily be explored using forceps to move the lung or by insufflating air into the pleural cavity to collapse it. Deep within the fissure are the hilum and the branches of the pulmonary artery which cannot be seen here. The perilobular veins are running through this lung section. Biopsies must not be taken in the fissures to avoid damaging these veins

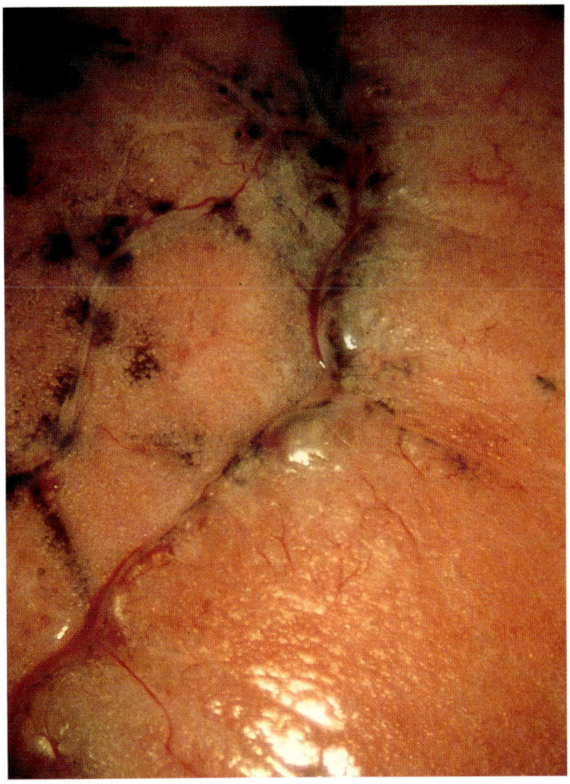

Fig. 19. Anthracotic pigment deposits and blebs. The amount of anthracotic pigment found in the lung is different in each patient. It is often distributed unevenly between the two lobes in the same patient. Here, the lower lobe presents moderate pigment deposits, outlining the pulmonary lobules which are approximately 1 cm in diameter. The upper lobe (on the *left)* is pinkish brown with no pigment. There are very small, shiny blebs on the edge of the fissure. This patient presented with a spontaneous pneumothorax. This type of lesion is found in almost every patient with spontaneous pneumothorax, when the lung is examined in detail. By contrast the ruptured bleb which caused the pneumothorax is rarely visible, as it has collapsed. It is understandable that in many cases of pneumothorax with such small lesions, patients do not suffer a relapse

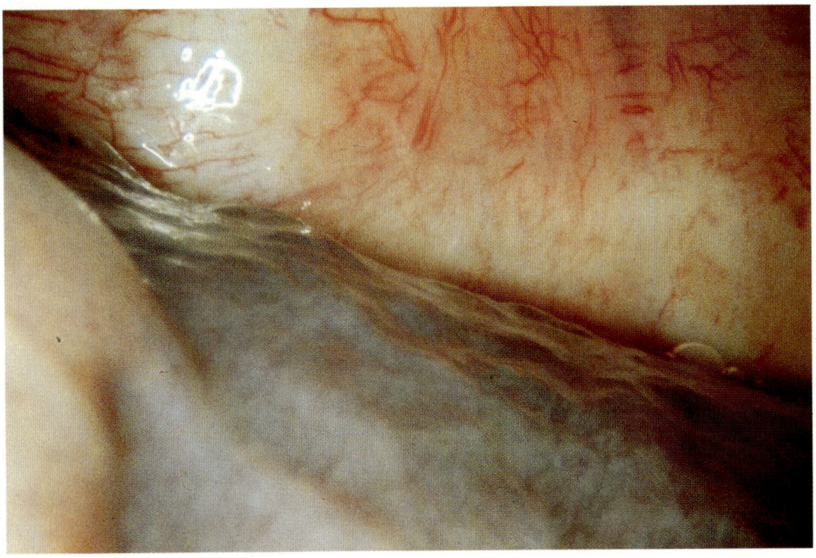

Fig. 20. Atelectasis. An atelectatic segment or lobe (here, the middle lobe) is easy to recognize; the collapsed area has a clear outline. It may be dark, violet-brown as shown above, or dark red or purplish in other cases

3.6.3 The Mediastinum and Great Vessels

The beginning thoracoscopist will best appreciate the normal endopleural anatomy while performing thoracoscopies in spontaneous pneumothorax. If the lung is gradually, gently compressed with insufflated air, it will retract to the hilum, allowing the inner thoracic organs to come into view.

On the left side (Figs. 21-22). A large artery can be seen quite distinctly, describing a concave infero-external curve: this is the subclavian artery, the easiest to locate and often the only one visible. It may or may not protrude into the pleural cavity; sometimes it appears to be almost detached from the mediastinum. Inferiorly, the subclavian artery is seen to originate from a large, pink, expansile vessel: the aortic arch. When touched with the thoracoscope, the intensity of the beat and the firmness of the aortic wall are distinctive. Further inferiorly, the lung partially covers the heart which can be seen from the front, however, by pushing the lung back with a probe or, with the help of gravity, by positioning the patient on his back. Pericardial abnormalities are visible from the left and biopsy of them is a simple matter. In cases of persistent pericardial effusion, a pericardial window can be created using Nd:YAG laser or electrocoagulation. Above and anterior to the subclavian artery, the left brachiocephalic venous trunk can be seen or at least made out; it hides the common carotid artery. The vagus and phrenic nerve are rarely visible, and the latter is seen more often on the right side. At the origin of the subclavian artery stands

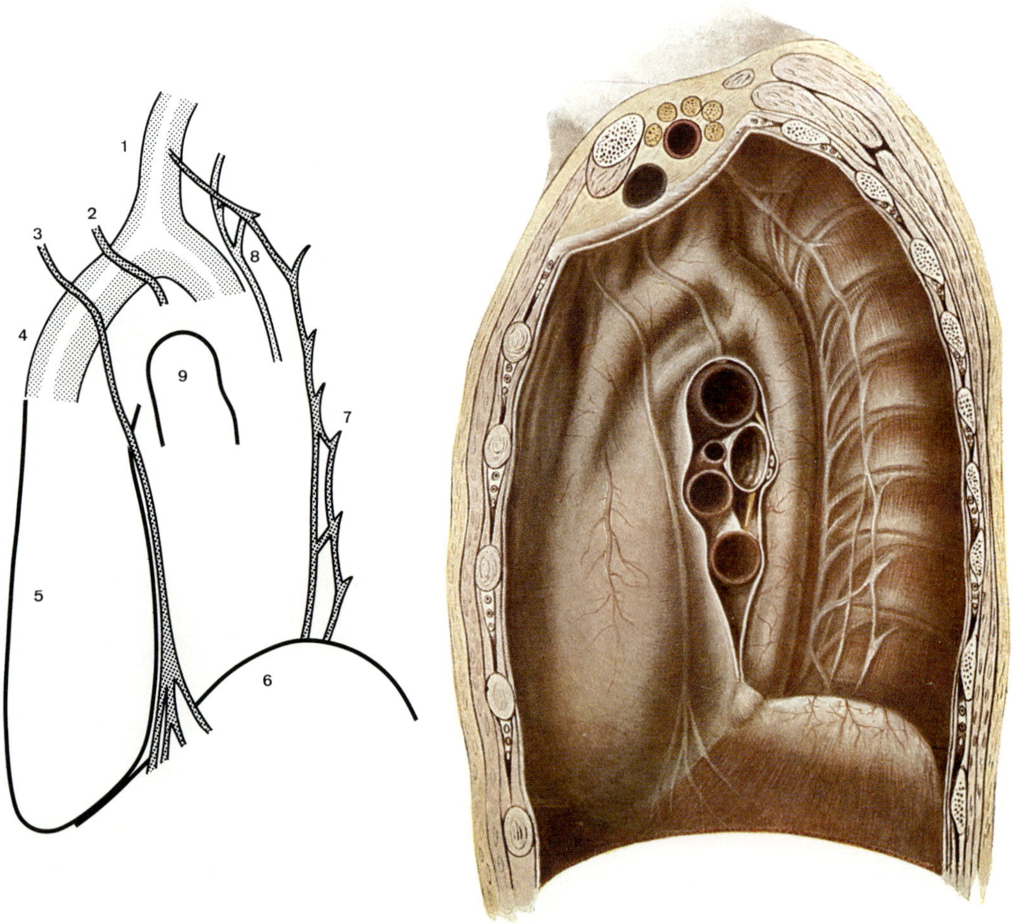

Fig. 21. The left pleural cavity. *1,* subclavian artery; *2,* vagus nerve; *3,* phrenic nerve; *4,* aortic arch; *5,* heart; *6,* diaphragm; *7,* sympathetic trunk; *8,* intercostal arteries and veins; *9,* hilum

a mid-mediastinal chain of lymph nodes that can be biopsied if necessary.

On the right side (Figs. 23, 69). The essential elements are the superior vena cava and the brachiocephalic (venous) trunk, with its junction with the subclavian vein just above. These veins are identified by their bluish color and their characteristic venous pulsations.

The phrenic nerve courses from the neck caudad over these great veins: it is easy to recognize because it resembles a white cord which stands out under the pleura which covers it. In one out of three cases, an accessory phrenic nerve anastomoses with it. At the top of the thorax, the phrenic nerve crosses the internal mammary artery and vein, located anteriorly and forming a cross which is easily visible in front of the superior vena cava, which the vein joins. Lower down, the nerve continues over the surface of the pericardium and can usually be followed down as far as the diaphragm.

The arterial brachiocephalic trunk (innominate artery) stands behind the upper portion of the phrenic nerve.

Lower down the azygos arch leads into the superior vena cava. It can easily be seen if the lung is collapsed. It is large, blue, pulsates, and runs in a posteroanterior direction.

The right auricle is situated under the hilum, crossed by the phrenic nerve; it has a soft consistency under the pericardium, and beats much less forcefully than the ventricles: its movement is very characteristic. Again, a biopsy of the pericardium from the right side is *strongly discouraged* since the wall of the auricle is very thin.

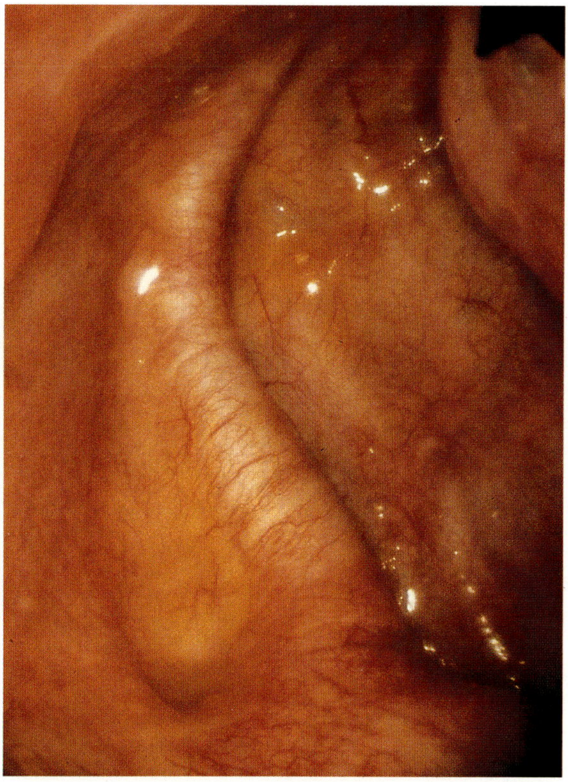

Fig. 22. The left pleural cavity. The subclavian artery runs upwards through the upper half of the left pleural cavity from the centre towards the outer edge. The aortic arch is clearly visible at the *bottom* of the photograph. Mediastinal fatty tissue, sometimes containing lymph nodes, can be seen to the left of the subclavian artery. The lung is situated on the *top right*. A large mediastinal vein often crosses in front of the subclavian artery, joining the innominate vein (brachiocephalic trunk). The hilum of the lung is situated just below the aortic arch. (See Fig. 69 for the right pleural cavity)

The trachea, with its identifying cartilaginous rings, is rarely visible. A depression can be seen behind the vena cava, where the vagus nerve travels from top to bottom and from front to back, and where the mid-mediastinal nodes can be accessed for thoracoscopic biopsy (Fig. 69).

On both sides. The internal mammary vessels protrude from the anterior wall and are seen along the entire length of the thorax.

The intercostal vessels are easily visible: the first four veins are grouped together to form the superior hemi-azygos on the left side and the superior root of the azygos on the right.

The diaphragm can easily be seen below, with its central tendon, muscles, and characteristic costal insertions.

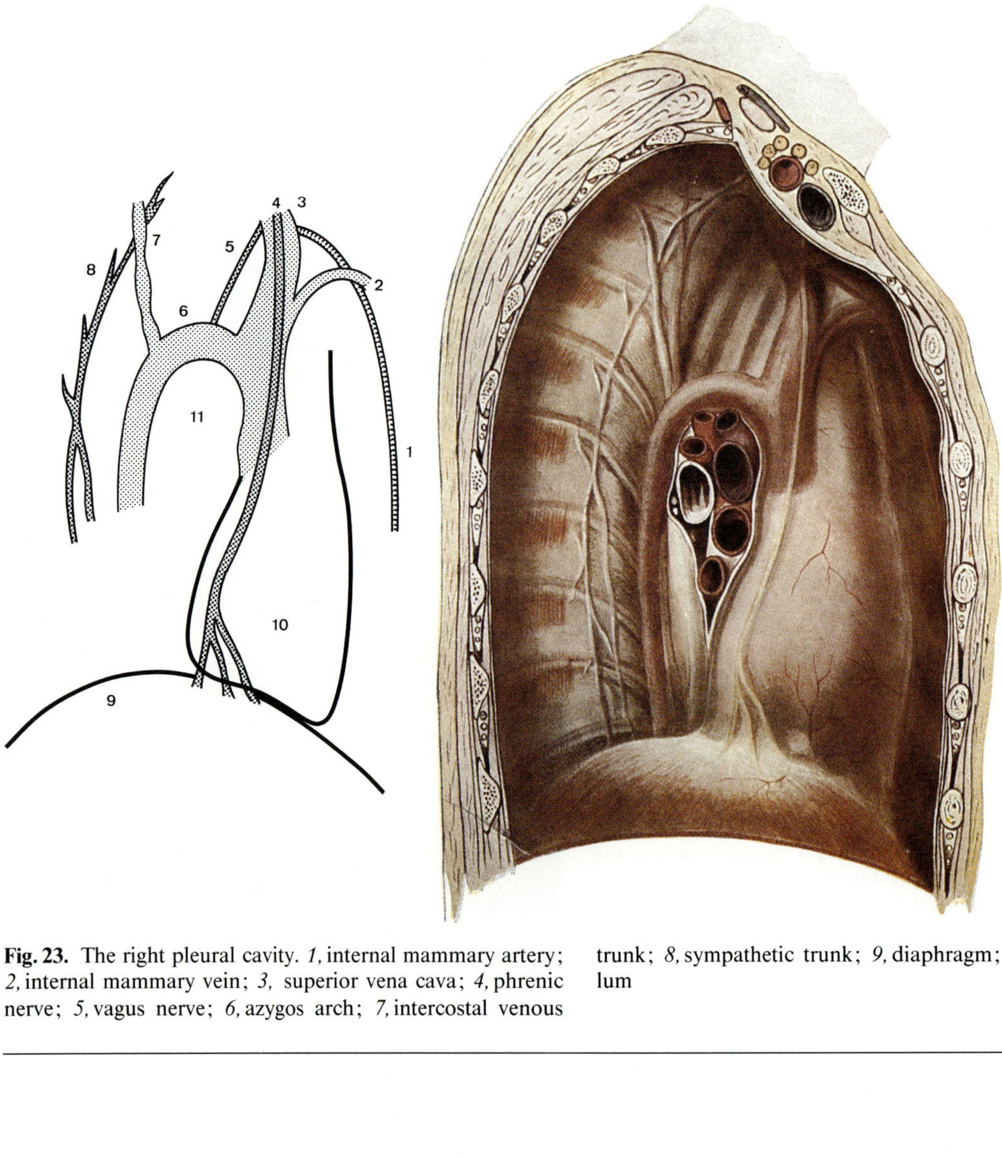

Fig. 23. The right pleural cavity. *1*, internal mammary artery; *2*, internal mammary vein; *3*, superior vena cava; *4*, phrenic nerve; *5*, vagus nerve; *6*, azygos arch; *7*, intercostal venous trunk; *8*, sympathetic trunk; *9*, diaphragm; *10*, heart; *11*, hilum

3.7 Pleural Biopsy Technique

Using optical forceps, pleural biopsies can be performed with a single point of entry. On the other hand, the 5-mm double spoon forceps, used with the dual entry approach, has the advantage of producing larger specimens, making the pathologist's investigations easier. When the pleura is thick, biopsy is a simple matter and there is no risk of cutting intercostal arteries or veins. By contrast, when the pleura is thin the biopsy should be performed against one of the ribs in order to eliminate the risk of bleeding from intercostal vessels. By touching the chest wall with the forceps it is easy to distinguish between the hard surface of bone and the spongy surface of the intercostal space (Fig. 24a).

In particular cases where the pleura is very hard and might tear when pulled by the forceps, some practitioners prefer to use HF instruments, which simultaneously cut the section and coagulate the biopsy site.

3.8 Number of Biopsies

Multiple large sections from different areas of the pleura must be submitted so that the pathologist has enough tissue for light microscopic examination and, if necessary, electron microscopy. Biopsy specimens may be submitted for immediate interpretation of frozen sections. However, pathologists are generally reluctant to commit themselves based on these preparations alone because pleural histology often appears quite different on the permanent sections. Indeed, distinguishing benign reactive mesothelial cells is difficult enough in fixed sections, and this difficulty is even greater with frozen sections. "Papanicolaou" cytologic smears of needle aspirates and brushings of the suspicious areas are more reliable (Bejui-Thivolet et al. 1984) (Fig. 24b).

Sufficient quantities of tissue for hormonal receptor assays can be obtained in cases of breast cancer or other hormone-dependent malignant tumors.

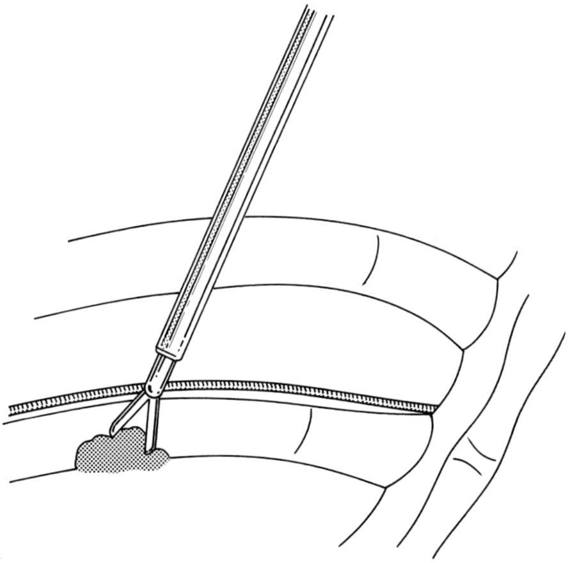

A

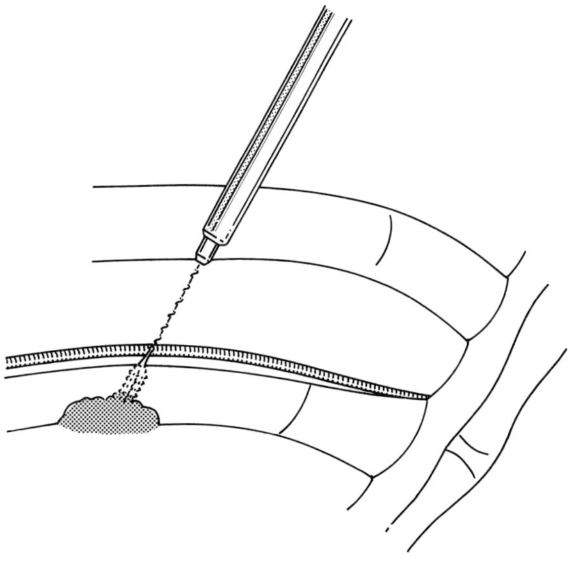

B

Fig. 24 A, B. Biopsy technique: the parietal pleura. **A** There are no serious problems when taking a biopsy of the parietal pleura. To avoid damaging the intercostal artery when the pleura is thin, the biopsy should be taken against the rib, so that the intercostal neurovascular bundle is not touched. **B** Endopleural brushings are easy to obtain under direct vision with the single entry-point technique. Here the brush is inserted through the trocar sheath using a 4-mm Panoview telescope

When the endoscopic picture is nonspecific, the total number of biopsies should be increased to 15–20, taken from the diaphragm, parietal pleura, costovertebral gutter, visceral pleura, etc., so that any still microscopic malignant tumor will not be missed (Morino et al. 1977). We believe that this large number of biopsies is necessary in order to fulfill one of the major goals of thoracoscopy, i. e., to confirm or eliminate a diagnosis of cancer with a high degree of certainty. This requires examination of many samples, which are carefully selected by the practitioner.

Special attention should be taken with fibrinous or necrotic deposits, as these can mask malignant lesions: they should be removed with forceps so that biopsies can be taken in their beds.

Since most lesions are found on the parietal pleura, multiple biopsies can rapidly be obtained. When the lesions are situated only on the visceral pleura, one or more pleuropulmonary biopsies are performed; bleeding is always minimal and any air leaks usually resolve promptly during the first few days postoperatively. To eliminate air leaks immediately the electrocautery instruments or YAG laser may be used.

Intercostal hemorrhaging is unusual and is never life-threatening when one or more of the following measures are taken: (a) tamponade of the bleeding site with an adrenalin-impregnated sponge; (b) coagulation using electrocautery or laser; (c) insertion of a chest tube with suction applied to bring the lung surface rapidly up against the chest wall. In our experience with over 1500 cases we have never had to call in a surgeon for hemorrhage or for any other reason.

3.9 The Second Point of Entry

Although a single point of entry is generally sufficient, in certain difficult situations a second point of entry can have major advantages and should be used in the following circumstances: (a) when movement of the trocar is sufficiently painful to the patient to limit access to an area of suspected abnormality. This may be due to simple geometric problems between the entry site and the lesion, or to a narrow intercostal space that limits the usual maneuverability of the in-

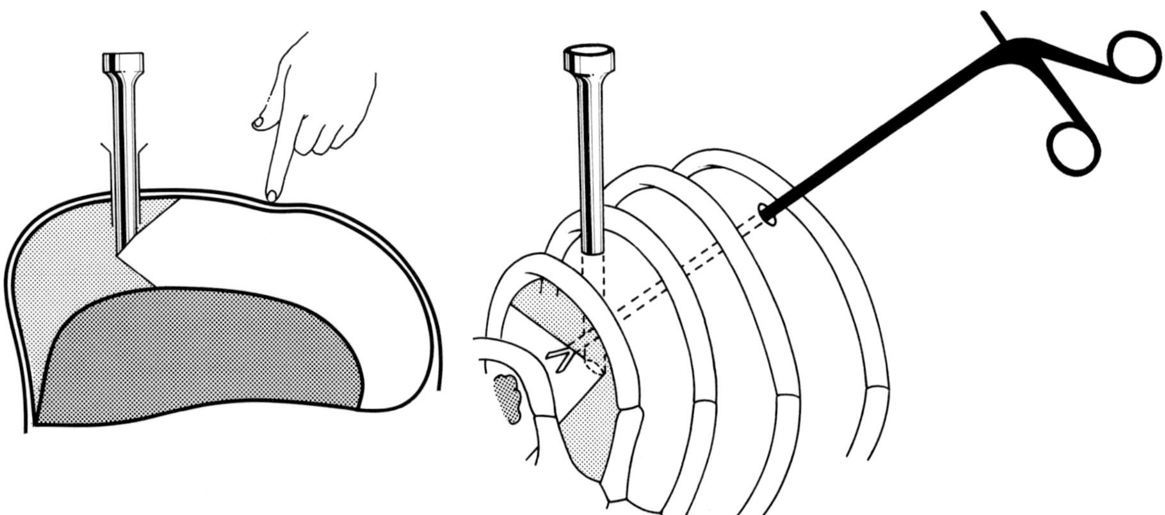

A B

Fig. 25 A, B. Exploration and biopsy using a 50° telescope: the second point of entry. **A** A telescope with a 50° angle of view allows the pleural cavity to be explored as if using an inverted periscope. A panoramic view is obtained by slowly rotating the telescope on its axis. This helps choose the best site for the second point of entry. **B** This telescope can also be used for selecting biopsy sites. 5 mm biopsy forceps is introduced through a second point of entry and directed to the biopsy site under visual control

struments. Although the local anesthetic provides excellent pain relief in the immediate area of entry, it has no effect on the ribs, which may experience pain if they are forcefully pushed up or down as the thoracoscope is rotated from its original position perpendicular to the chest wall to a more acute angle; (b) when there are large adhesions, making it necessary to either divide them or circumvent them; (c) when a thorough inspection of the entire pleura from the apex and the superior mediastinum down to the diaphragm is desired; (d) when electrocautery or laser is to be used in conjunction with pleural or, especially, pulmonary biopsies.

The second point of entry is established quickly and easily. Its position is determined by viewing through the 50° scope while depressing the possible entry site with the index finger (Fig. 25 a): the resulting endopleural depression can easily be seen. Sometimes it is helpful to actually insert a needle through that same site while viewing its precise location through the thoracoscope.

After administering local anesthetic, a 5-mm incision is made and the 5-mm trocar is directly inserted. This trocar will accomodate many instruments designed for its smaller bore, including the 4-mm Panoview with either lateral or direct optical telescope, double-spoon biopsy forceps equipped for electrocautery (Fig. 25 B), laser fiber, and a loop for dividing adhesions.

3.10 Dividing Adhesions (Pneumonolysis) (Figs. 26 A, B; 28)

Fibrinous adhesions in the form of threads, cords, or veils cannot usually be seen on routine roentgenograms and may still go undetected on X-rays taken after induced pneumothorax. They may therefore come as a surprise to the inexperienced physician. Generally, they are easy to divide and may break apart immediately when grasped with forceps. Otherwise, a brief application of HF current (or laser) will divide them.

If the adhesion is thick, a second point of entry is selected so that the adhesion can be approached perpendicularly (Figs. 26 A, 26 B). It is sectioned using forceps or a diathermy loop by winding it around the instrument while the physician pulls it towards himself. This increases the contact area, makes coagulation easier, and avoids any risk of hemorrhage. Coagulation should take place as far as possible from the lung surface, close to the parietal pleura, starting at the back and moving forwards slowly in a step-by-step approach. Avoid the large vessels which are found in the mediastinum and the apex of the thoracic cage. During electrocauterization, the adhesion increases in size to form a rim of white necrotic tissue around the section.

Adhesions can interfere with the procedure in at least three situations where it is important to cut them off: (a) when a veil of adhesions hinders exploration of an important part of the pleural cavity; (b) when a pulmonary breach which created a pneumothorax is held open by an adjacent adhesion, thus perpetuating the pneumothorax; or (c) when an adhesion is in close contact with a suspected malignant pulmonary lesion. After biopsying the lung, the adhesion might hold the biopsy breach open, leading to an enduring broncho-pleural fistula (the biopsy should be avoided if the adhesion can not be divided).

In summary, it should be emphasized that dividing major adhesions is generally unnecessary and the beginning thoracoscopist need not con-

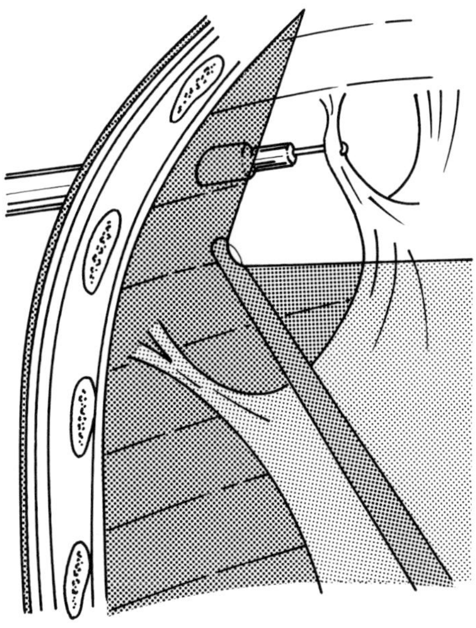

Fig. 26 A. Lysis of adhesions (pneumonolysis). Here, the coagulating loop is positioned using a 50° Panoview telescope

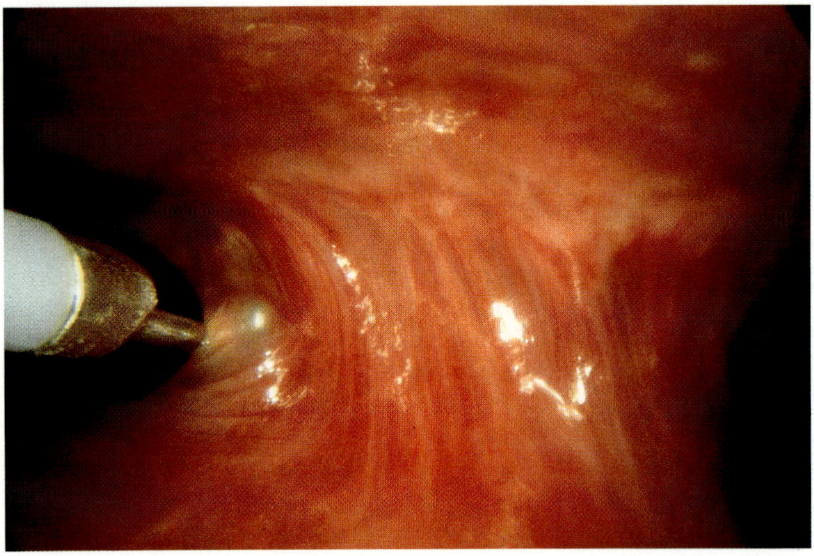

Fig. 26B. Severing large adhesions. Large adhesions are severed gradually using an electrocautery loop, starting at one end of the adhesion; here, its left side. The adhesion should be separated using the hook; the operator pulls the area to be sectioned towards himself until the end of the loop can be seen. This ensures that the lung is not damaged in the process

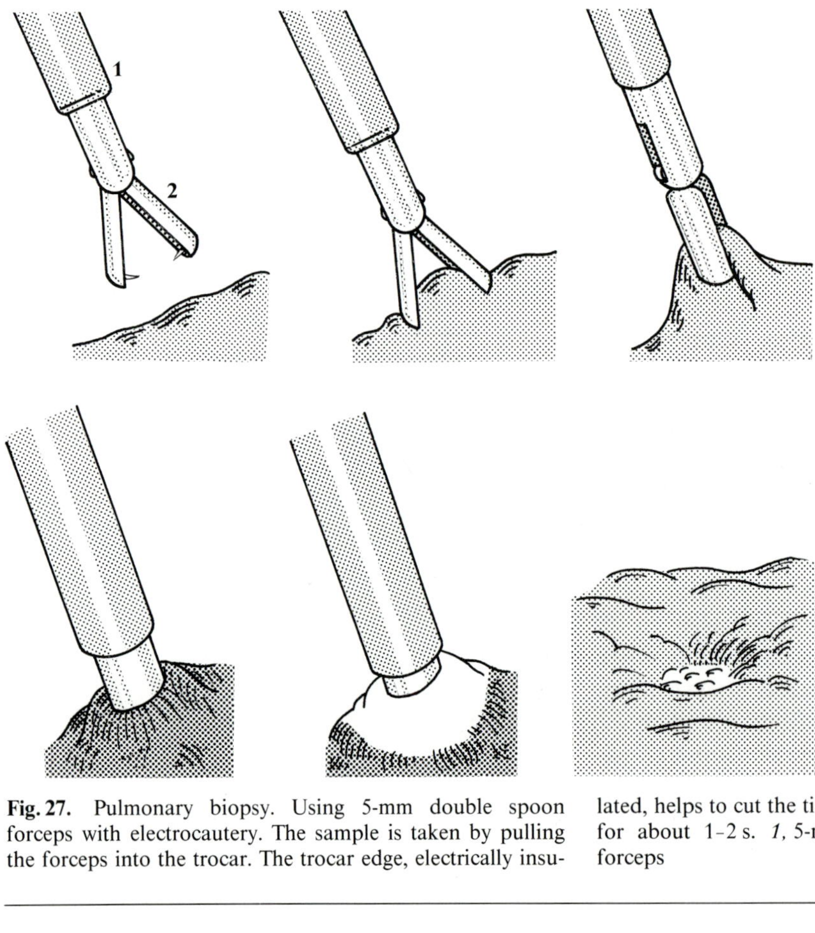

Fig. 27. Pulmonary biopsy. Using 5-mm double spoon forceps with electrocautery. The sample is taken by pulling the forceps into the trocar. The trocar edge, electrically insulated, helps to cut the tissue while electrocautery is turned on for about 1–2 s. *1*, 5-mm trocar sheath; *2*, double spoon forceps

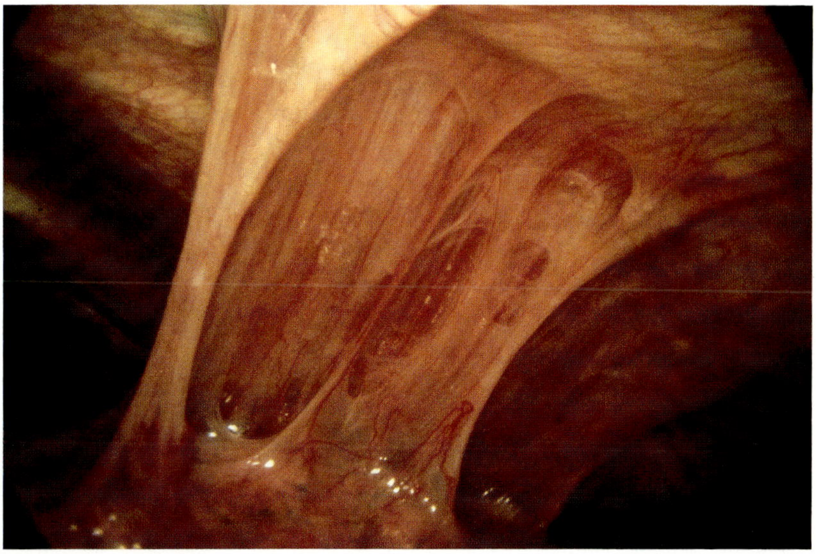

Fig. 28. Inflammatory adhesions. Some adhesions are thin, almost transparent. Vessels may be seen running along their length. The adhesions should be cut close to the ribs to avoid damaging the lung. They are divided using a laser or an electrocautery loop to ensure hemostasis of the vessels. Adhesions like these are often found in recurrent spontaneous pneumothorax along the pathway of an anterior chest tube; they do not bind the lung tightly enough to the chest wall to prevent relapses

cern himself greatly about this problem. Significantly interfering adhesions which resist simple probing and forceps removal are sufficiently infrequent and therefore relegate the technique of pneumonolysis to a secondary role in modern thoracoscopy.

3.11 The Pulmonary Biopsy Technique (Figs. 27, 29, 30)

Biopsies are performed using coagulating forceps on a medium setting of approximately 100 W. We recommend to first select the best setting by testing it on animals, or simply on a piece of meat. An intensity is chosen which will coagulate the cut surface of the lung without destroying the histologic features of the specimen taken with a 5-mm double-spoon forceps.

The practitioner holds the direct or oblique-angle telescope in one hand and the coagulating forceps in the other (Fig. 29). The assistant holds the trocar cannulas firmly in place as previously indicated.

Probing the lung with forceps helps to locate suspected areas. Tumors are much firmer than the usually soft lung; they may have a red or white tint and can be either raised (pleural metastases) or umbilicated (pulmonary metastases). One should note the vascularity, its consistency, and whether or not there are adjacent adhesions to be freed. Diathermy settings may require adjustment within the previously established range.

The biopsy area is grasped with the forceps perpendicular to the pulmonary surface. Close the forceps for 1–2 seconds, then pull them towards the 5-mm trocar; apply current briefly (approximately one second) using a foot pedal, while pulling the forceps through the distal end of the trocar which will help to cut the section (Fig. 27). In our experience, the dry weight of lung biopsies has ranged from 4 to 37 mg.

After each sample has been taken, the biopsy site blanches and retracts slightly. It does not bleed and looks uniform, with no evident air leak (Fig. 30).

We generally take one to eight biopsies in a given session. Healthy-looking areas as well as abnormal ones should be biopsied. It is not unusual for an area that is endoscopically abnormal to contain nonspecific fibrosis on biopsy, while relatively normal-looking tissue at the periphery of the lesion yields specific diagnostic information.

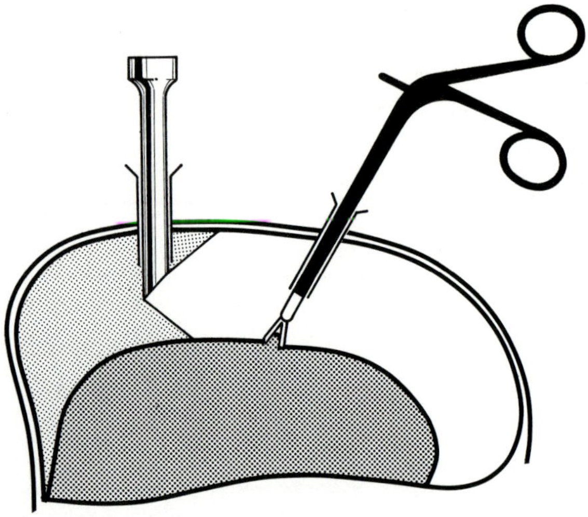

Fig. 29 A. Pulmonary biopsy using two points of entry. Pulmonary biopsy under direct vision using a 50° telescope. If the second point of entry is to be a long way from the first (at about 4 to 5 fingers' width), the cannula is positioned so that the forceps are directed straight towards the area to be biopsied

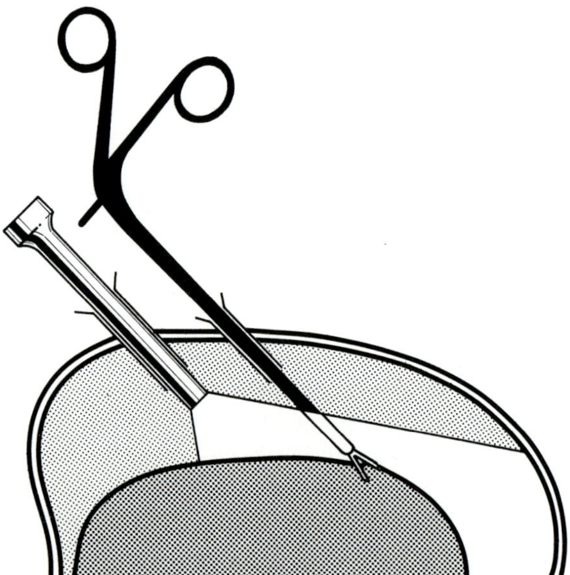

Fig. 29 B. Pulmonary biopsy under direct vision using a 0° telescope. The physician who is new to the technique will find it easier to work with the instruments parallel to each other, about 3 to 4 cm apart. The telescope is held in the left hand and the biopsy forceps in the right, keeping them parallel. This technique is in fact more limited than the one above, as the 50° telescope has a wider field of view

Never perform biopsies in the fissures, since they may contain large mediastinal and fissural veins.

Emphysematous bullae and cavities in a honeycomb lung should systematically be avoided, since biopsy may lead to prolonged air leak after the procedure. As emphysematous bullae often occur at the base of the lung, random biopsies are preferentially taken from the mid- or upper-lung regions.

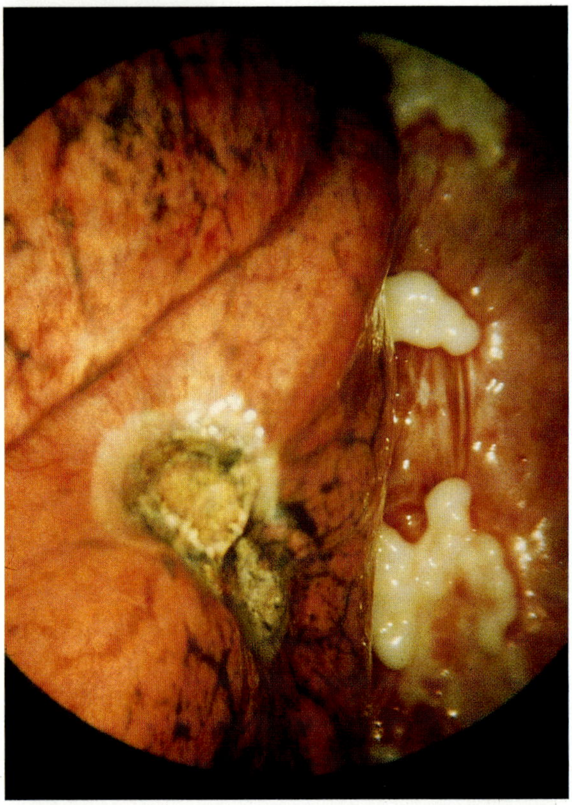

Fig. 30. Pulmonary biopsy. This patient, formerly exposed to asbestos, presented with asbestotic, fibrohyaline pleural plaques. Note that these plaques are situated exclusively on the parietal pleura, and that the lung appears normal. As all sputum tests for ferruginous bodies were negative, two pulmonary biopsies were taken: one for pathological diagnosis of asbestosis and one for an asbestos fiber count under an electronic microscope, using Sebastien's technique (Boutin et al. 1981 c). This sample contained 19×10^6 amphibole fibers and 6.7×10^6 chrysotile fibers per gram of dry pulmonary tissue. Coagulating forceps were used to ensure hemostasis and aerostasis of the lung: one can see the biopsy scar in the *center* of the photograph. Several biopsies can be taken from different areas. Chest tube drainage brings the lung back to its position against the chest wall. The drain is usually removed on the third day

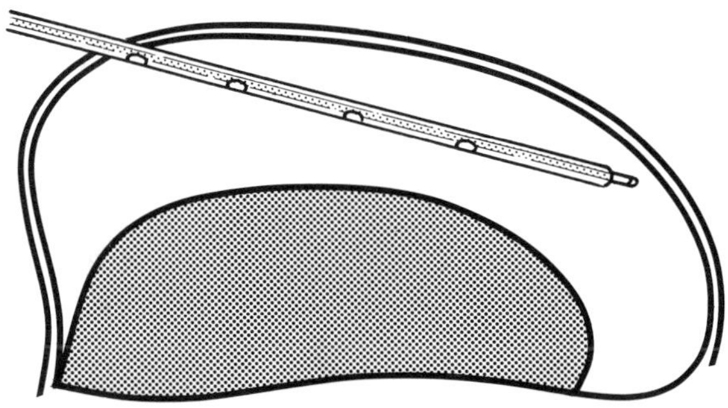

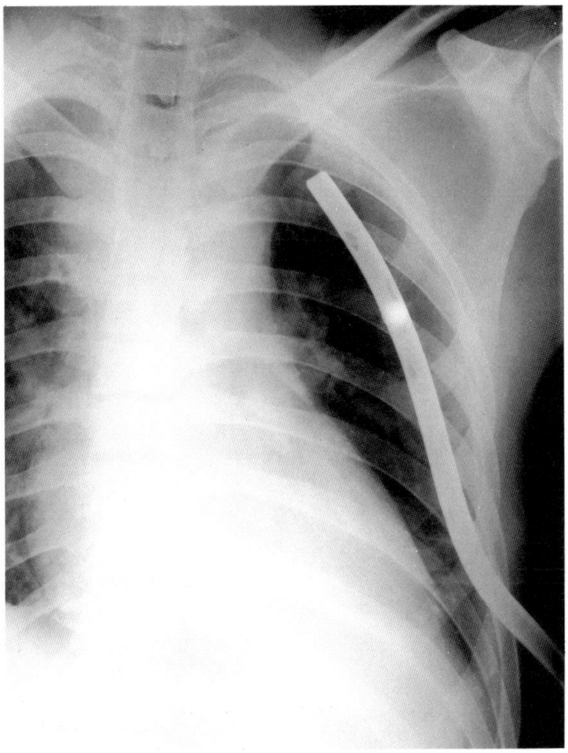

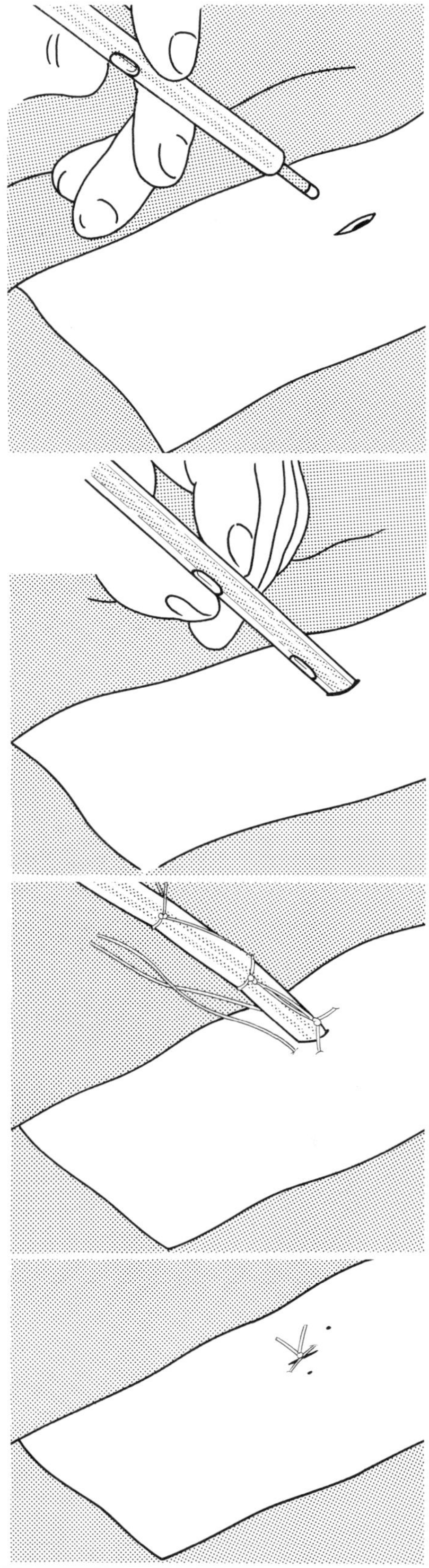

Fig. 31. Chest tube placement using a blunt inner trocar. The blunt inner trocar allows the drainage tube to be inserted through the thoracoscopy incision and to be positioned atraumatically high in the cavity. The chest tube is tied to the skin. A purse-string suture is placed, in anticipation of closing the incision when the chest tube is removed

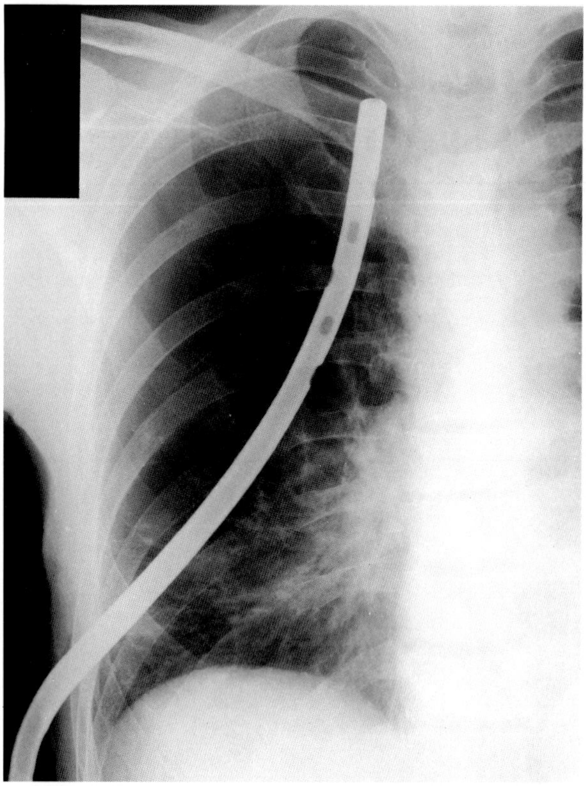

A

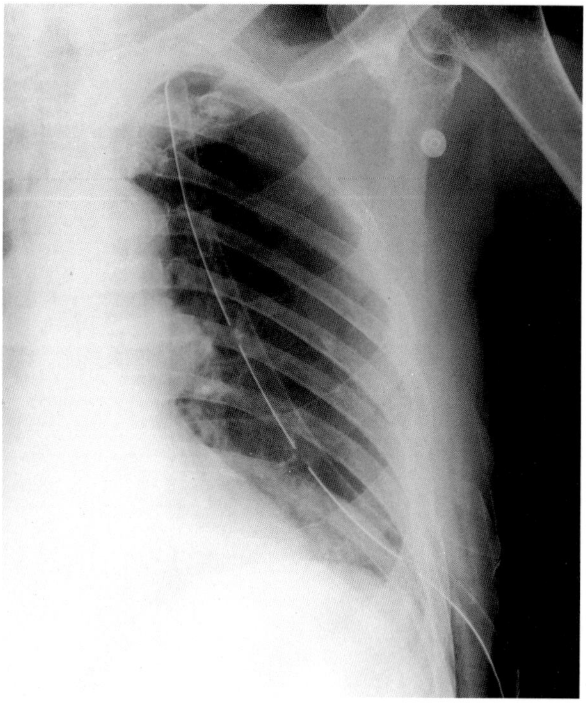

B

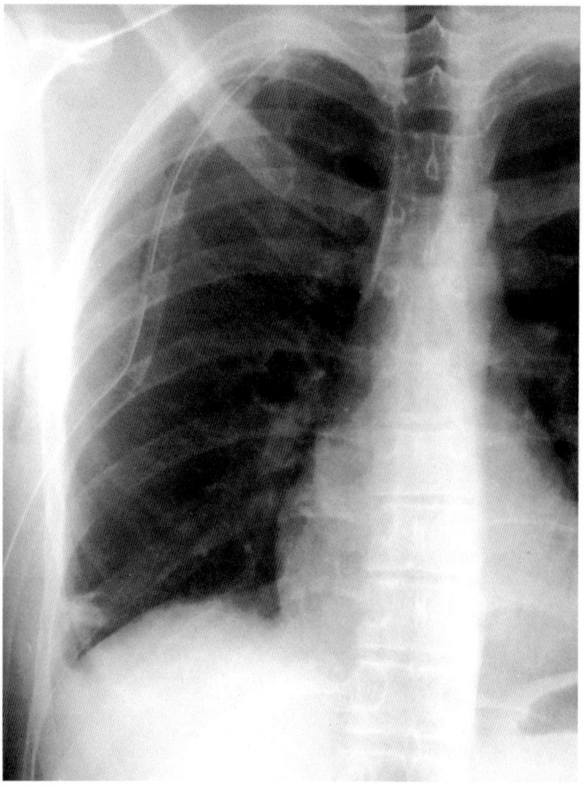

C

Fig. 32 A–C. Pleural drainage: various positions of the tube. **A** A 30 Fr rubber tube may be used in case of spontaneous pneumothorax after talc has been used. Here, the tube is inserted in the 6th intercostal space. It is always positioned high in the cavity, **B** A 28 Fr plastic tube is used in case of pleurisy after talc poudrage. The tube is positioned high in the pleural cavity and is inserted in the 7th intercostal space, so that all the fluid is drained, **C** A 28 Fr plastic drain for use in a chronic pneumothorax when talc has been used. The drain is inserted in the 2nd intercostal space on the midclavicular line, and is positioned high in the cavity

3.12 The Rest of the Examination

Inspecting the pleura and performing biopsies are the two essential steps of the examination. Complementary endopleural photography or videotaping may be helpful later on, especially in difficult cases where biopsies proved nondiagnostic, in occupational diseases where direct visual review of gross pathology may be more impressive than the physician's description of it, and in teaching institutions. The experienced thoracoscopist quickly becomes accustomed to looking at the video screen instead of the ocular of the thoracoscope.

When inspection and biopsy have been completed, talc poudrage is often performed to promote pleurodesis in the treatment of chronic, recurrent pleural effusions or spontaneous pneumothorax (see Sect. 6.4).

3.13 Positioning the Chest Tube for Pleural Drainage (Figs. 31–33)

At the end of thoracoscopy, a chest tube is inserted through the point of entry. When a small tube is sufficient (18 Fr), it can be inserted through the cannula and guided to the required area. However, it is not always possible to aim it in the best direction, especially if there are many adhesions. In addition, we have obtained more complete drainage results using a 24–32 Fr tube mounted on a 50-cm blunt guide and inserted immediately after removing the trocar canula. The tube is pushed through the point of entry, perpendicular to the skin at first, then pointed in the desired direction until it meets the chest wall. No special force is required.

Ideally, the tube is directed posteriorly and then as close to the apex as possible. Since this may leave the tube holes high in the thorax, fluid drainage may be improved by making one or two extra holes on the radio-opaque side of the inferior part of the tube (Fig. 31); make sure, however, that the proximal hole will remain 1–2 cm from the internal orifice of the chest wall. Aspiration of the remaining fluid and air generally requires only a few minutes. When thoracoscopy is performed for diagnosis of a pleural effusion, the tube may be quickly removed as soon as the effectiveness of the maneuver is confirmed radiographically. In other cases, the tube is left in place for several days, either until drainage provides less than 100 ml of fluid per day after talc poudrage (usually 2–3 days); or until all bubbling ceases after lung biopsy or treatment for pneumothorax (seldom more than 3–4 days).

When the chest tube is to be left in place for drainage, a simple suture is applied to secure it firmly to the skin. An additional purse-string suture is placed while the local anesthetic is still

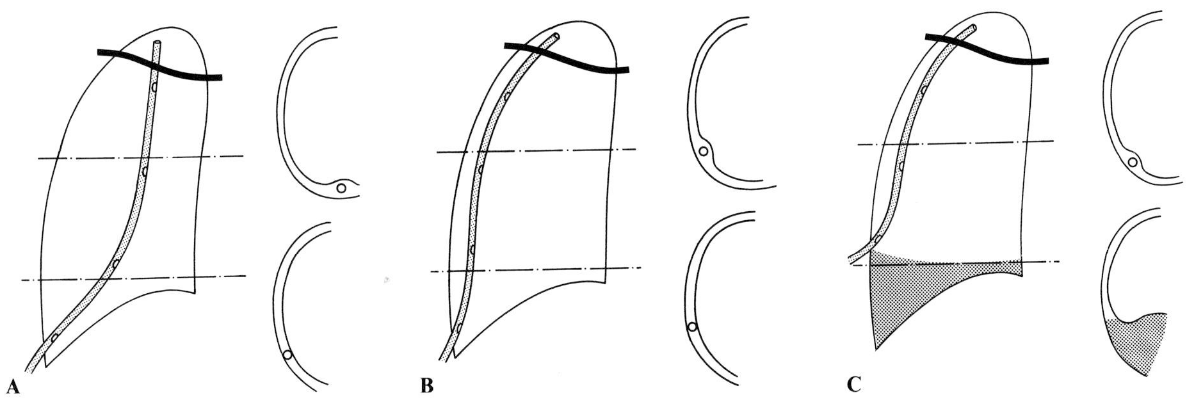

Fig. 33 A–C. Pleural fluid drainage: positioning the chest tube. **A** The tube is placed in the costovertebral gutter: the posterior part of the pleural space is efficiently drained. **B** Placing the tube in an axillary position may hinder drainage of the posterior part of the pleura. **C** Fluid may collect below the tube if it is inserted too high. **A** is better than **B**; both are better than **C**

effective. The purse string is left open until tube removal, when it is tightly tied to close the chest wall wound. Wound healing allows this suture to be removed after another 7-10 days.

3.14 The YAG Laser Option

When the endoscopy room is equipped with a YAG laser, its use in thoracoscopy is of interest. It does not usually require special equipment, although one can use a thoracoscope that is specially adapted for the laser fiber, allowing introduction through a single point of entry (Fig. 2G; Boutin 1986b, 1989a).

3.14.1 Materials

A special thoracoscope, manufactured by Wolf and equipped with a Panoview telescope (diameter: 4 mm, angle: 25°), gives a wide angle of view. Continuous videotape recording makes it possible to view enlarged images and to work without having to wear special glasses during laser usage.

A second point of entry may also be used. In this case, the fiber goes through a sheath, a simple metal cylinder of 4 mm in diameter and 20 cm in length. The physician holds the thoracoscope in one hand and the fiber in the other which is then directed as desired.

The length and intensity of the laser beam can be set according to indications. We use an intensity of 30-50 W with visual verification. During the procedure, obstruction of the cannula must be avoided in order to enable the vapor and smoke to freely leave the thorax during respiratory movements. The action of the laser is instantaneous and does not really prolong the examination.

One can operate under selective intubation of the opposite lung. Thus, immobilizing the laser-treated lung minimizes the chance of injury to it.

3.14.2 Indications

Pulmonary biopsies. The laser can be used, after biopsy with forceps, to ensure airtightness of the lung: after removing samples of pulmonary parenchyma, the laser fiber is introduced and the pulmonary orifice is closed by 3-5 laser pulses. Closure is immediate: one observes a shrinkage of the lung around the biopsy hole, ensuring both hemostasis and aerostasis (Figs. 70A, B).

The physician should keep in mind that the laser beam will penetrate the parenchyma to a depth that varies with the intensity setting; for a setting of approximately 30-40 W, this depth will vary from 5 to 10 mm. The laser should therefore be stopped as soon as the desired result has been obtained.

Adhesions. When the lysis of adhesions is indicated, the laser can do an excellent job. It ensures hemostasis of the section, is efficient, rapid, and does not present any technical difficulty.

Closure of Pulmonary Orifices. A small pulmonary wound can easily be coagulated by laser. We have used this technique in the following conditions:

(a) in certain cases of pneumothorax by acupuncture where the pulmonary wound was therefore minimal, (b) in two cases of pneumothorax provoked by an unfortunate attempt to catheterize the subclavian vein, and (c) in a case of traumatic hemopneumothorax by knife wound. We also coagulated, from the interior, bleeding in the intercostal space.

Pleuropulmonary fistulae with empyema. We have tried to use the laser for this pathology but the results have been poor. In two cases we obtained a good result by associating a decortication by laser of the fistula edges and pleural talcage followed by drainage. In another case, we used 2 ml of biological glue (Tissucol). In three other cases, these maneuvers failed because the fistulae were too large.

The problem posed by bronchopleural fistulae is often dramatic, with death ensuing in 30%-50% of the patients with cancers. Several unfavorable factors should be emphasized. The purulence of the pleurisy, the cancerous nature of the underlying condition, malnutrition with emaciation, muscular wasting and severe protein deficiency, and resistance of the microbes to antibiotics. All of these factors together result in the fact that straightforward laser-induced obliteration of the fistula is not always possible especially without management of malnutrition and the infectious processes; even if the lung were cauterized and the orifice temporarily closed, the persisting infection and malnutrition would rapidly cause the fistula to reopen.

Spontaneous Pneumothorax. We have carried out the cauterization of emphysematous bullae or blebs in 30 patients. In some cases there were bullae or blebs in the apex, isolated or grouped together, less than or equal to 1.5–2 cm in size. Other patients presented with small superficial blebs of a few millimeters in diameter which were easily coagulated. Finally, in other cases, the visceral pleura was abnormal, dull, and easily split from the pulmonary parenchyma if seized by forceps. We coagulated the abnormal areas by using the laser once every square centimeter or so.

We obtained very good immediate results in all cases except one. There was one case of recurrence after 18 months of follow-up.

When endoscopic lesions are visible and generally limited to the apex, their destruction by laser would seem to be justified: in any case, a surgeon would do the same thing, but with thoracoscopy, thoracotomy is avoided. The problem is different if the lesions are diffuse; either the bullae are very large and it is better to send the patient to a surgeon, or the lesions are small but very numerous and one can coagulate the larger ones and resort to medical pleurodesis for the others.

3.15 Conclusion

The physician must be committed to performing a complete and rapid thoracoscopic examination. To ensure this, one must carefully plan all activities and whenever possible make the following decisions ahead of time:

1. Choose the point of entry using X-rays taken after induced pneumothorax in order to locate the regions most likely to be biopsied.
2. Estimate the need for biopsies of pleura and diaphragm as well as lung.
3. Prepare labels for the pathologist and cytologist so that samples may be promptly submitted to the appropriate technical personnel. (Whenever possible, more specific information regarding the exact location of the biopsy site should be added at the time of sampling).
4. Anticipate the need for special preservative solutions or for special handling of biopsies for mineralogic analysis (dust-free 10% formalin), hormone receptor assays, special microbiologic studies (mycobacterial, mycologic, viral, anaerobic, etc.), electron microscopy, or tissue culture.

It is, therefore, impossible to carry out a complete, effective, and high-yield thoracoscopy without high level laboratory backup to handle the specimens; a good working relationship with the laboratory staff can be a decisive factor. Fortunately, most major hospitals today have the essential scientific capabilities to provide this level of support.

Chapter 4: Thoracoscopic Sequelae: Side Effects, Complications, Prevention

Thoracoscopic sequelae are infrequently a problem. Those problems that do occur, however, were well known to earlier phthisiologists, who recorded them in their texts (Dumarest et al. 1914, 1954; Alexander 1937). The most common complaints are dyspnea, cough, and pain which occurs primarily during biopsy and electrocoagulation, or is due to pressure on the ribs. Vagal syncope has been described. More dramatic is subcutaneous emphysema or, rarely, mediastinal emphysema which has occasionally been fatal (Douady and Meyer 1942). These emphysematous complications have been eliminated by inserting a simple chest drainage tube at the end of the procedure.

Douady and Meyer have mentioned the possibility of sudden death just from induction of pneumothorax. Air embolism has also been reported, but this occurred primarily when the procedure was carried out in the sitting position.

The patient's temperature sometimes rises slightly (up to 38°C) after thoracoscopy, but it very rarely indicates a superinfection of the pleural space due to failure of antiseptic techniques (De Camp et al. 1973).

These occurrences were infrequent in the past – although some surgeons, who were critical of phthisiologists, dwelled on them – and they are extremely rare at present. Modern thoracoscopy has evolved to become an usually safe procedure. Viskum (1981, 1989a) found only one fatality in his review of 8000 examinations. Of the 4301 cases we have culled from the literature (Boutin et al. 1982b, 1984), the death rate was only 0.09%, which is impressively low compared to thoracotomy or any other pulmonary endoscopic examination (Wall et al. 1981).

However, the safety of the procedure depends on one's mastery of the technique and upon careful observation of the patient, as in any pleural drainage procedure. The physician must take a number of precautions which we have learned through experience and will enumerate below.

4.1 Morbidity

Our earliest experience was gained prior to 1978. We gradually improved our technique while using a single point of entry on 200 patients, first with a 12-mm thoracoscope and then a 10-mm laparoscope with a central operating channel, allowing a 3-mm biopsy forceps to be inserted but not an electrocoagulating device. Pneumonolysis was impossible using this equipment. As with Viskum, we did not routinely leave a pleural drainage tube postoperatively. Using these methods, our diagnostic yield in malignant diseases was only 78% (Boutin et al. 1981a). This low yield coupled with two perioperative deaths led us to question the overall efficacy of thoracoscopy and to review the associated morbidity we experienced:

1. Two cases of major hemorrhage after intercostal biopsies: these totalled 500 ml and 1500 ml of blood in 24 h; both were treated with blood transfusion, and spontaneously ceased without recourse to surgical intervention.
2. Four cases of minor parietal pleural bleeding of less than 50 ml.
3. Two mild episodes of hemoptysis caused by endotracheal intubation.
4. One case of right lung atelectasis (which actually was due to a malignant endobronchial mass occluding the right main bronchus).
5. One superinfection of the pleural space, which

occurred during postoperative chest tube drainage.
6. One case of "pleural shock" with trembling, tachycardia, and cardiovascular collapse.
7. Four cases of extensive subcutaneous emphysema, one of which also had mediastinal emphysema leading to death a few hours after the examination. (We had made the mistake of not leaving a chest tube at the end of the procedure.)
8. One other death occurred 15 min after the procedure due to acute reexpansion pulmonary edema. The lung had been rapidly reexpanded under too negative a pressure. This was a known cardiac patient with generalized cancer.
9. One other death in a terminal cancer patient occurred 5 days after thoracoscopy, but in this case death was deemed unrelated to the operation.

As a result of this mortality and morbidity review and because of our disappointment with the 78% yield in cancer patients, we revised our technique in 1978 and applied some preventive measures enumerated in Chap. 3. We also seriously reviewed the morbidity reported by others, such as Douady and Meyer:

Pulmonary perforations were seen as a result of careless introduction of the pleural trocar, easily avoidable with prudence; or with too hasty or forceful tugging on thick adhesions; or as a consequence of pulmonary biopsy. Although these perforations with associated air leaks were widely feared in the past, experience in the last 20-30 years has shown that water-seal drainage permits the defect to heal without serious respiratory compromise, usually within a few days. We found the application of negative pressure to the chest tube to be generally unhelpful in this context: indeed, suction at times may perpetuate a pleural breach by holding the edges in the open position and preventing their reapposition. As for a theoretical "scab loss" that could follow coagulation of the lung surface, producing a broncho-pleural fistula, its very existence has always been controversial, and we have never observed it.

Cardiac incidents are mostly self-limited: tachyarrhythmia, hypotension, transitory myocardial ischemia.

Finally, it is important to note a complication of thoracoscopy which is not rare in malignant pleural disease, especially mesothelioma: contamination of the entry tract with tumor cells, followed by growth of the tumor itself within this tract (Blanchette et al. 1973; Elmes and Simpson 1976; Miech et al. 1967; Migueres and Jover 1975b). This complication may even be seen after a simple thoracentesis or pleural needle biopsy (Boutin et al. 1975b; Miech et al. 1967). At any rate, serious growth at the needle or thoracoscope entry site can be prevented easily, as will be discussed in a later section (4.2.3).

Overall, these complications are rare today and are listed in large measure because an understanding of them will enable the thoracoscopist to avoid them.

4.2 Practical Preventive Measures

Thoracoscopy is thus a simple technique which can be performed by any chest physician with a certain amount of dexterity, as long as some basic rules are respected.

4.2.1 Criteria for Patient Selection

We use the following absolute requirements for the procedure: arterial blood gas: $pO2 > 50$ torr while breathing room air.
Coagulation:
Prothrombin time $> 60\%$
Cephalin-kaolin time $> 70\%$
Platelet count > 70000/cubic-mm.
Otherwise, there are only a few *absolute contraindications* to thoracoscopy. The principal one is insufficient space in the pleural cavity: the minimum space required for insertion of a thoracoscope is approximately 10 cm in diameter. Furthermore, the lesion must be within the accessible area. If roentgenograms suggest that the lesion is outside the area of the pneumothorax, it is generally best not to attempt conventional

thoracoscopy. (Alternatives in this situation include thoracotomy or the direct thoracoscopic technique developed by Maassen, 1981, which does not require pneumothorax; see p. 4).

As a matter of common sense, absolute contraindications to pulmonary biopsy also include: (a) honeycomb lung: there is a high risk of persistent air leak and, in any case, the pathologist will predictably find excess collagen deposition without specific diagnostic features, (b) pulmonary arteriovenous aneurysms, (c) suspected hydatid cysts, and (d) highly vascularized pulmonary lesions.

Relative contraindications concern the general health of the patient, and a careful risk/benefit analysis at the time thoracoscopy is considered. Fever, cough, hypoxemia, hypocoagulable state, unstable cardiovascular status, etc., may all prevent the procedure, although the contraindication is almost always temporary.

Temporary contraindications lead to postponement of thoracoscopy until a safer time. Temperature should be normal and the patient free of infection, unless the examination is being performed for diagnosis or treatment of empyema.

Refractory cough is avoided because of the high risk of subcutaneous emphysema and of increased pain at the chest tube site; furthermore, the high intrabronchial pressures create a serious risk for persistent air leak after pulmonary biopsy.

Hypocoagulability may often be corrected by fresh plasma, platelet transfusions, vitamin K, etc. Heart failure and hypoxemia may often be improved with time and medical management.

4.2.2 Patient Monitoring During the Examination

The pulse, blood pressure, and respiration are carefully monitored. Depending on the equipment available, local custom, and the patient's clinical condition, electrocardiographic and continuous pulse oximetry monitoring are used. Oxygen is administered as required.

Hemorrhages caused by injury to a parietal vessel during biopsy (Rodgers 1981) are extremely rare and can be avoided, as already described, by making sure that the lesion being biopsied is supported by something hard underneath, such as the ribs (see p. 31).

To avoid subcutaneous emphysema at the end of thoracoscopy, all intrapleural air should be aspirated and the lung reexpanded against the chest wall. Pleural drainage must routinely be completed.

The lung is reexpanded gently, without strong negative pressures, to avoid any risk of pulmonary edema.

Of course, aseptic conditions, must be maintained at all times.

4.2.3 Local Preventive Radiotherapy (Fig. 34)

In cases of mesothelioma, local preventive radiotherapy is carried out routinely to destroy malignant cells seeded in the puncture tract: 10–12 days after thoracoscopy, once the incision has healed, we apply electron therapy, between 12.5 and 15 MeV, to the thoracic wall, penetrating to an average depth of 3 cm, by giving 21 Gy in 48 h (3 sessions of 7 Gy). The irradiated field is approximately 10 cm on a side, centered over the healing wound and over all puncture sites from previous thoracenteses. A 1-cm thick paraffin plaque brings the isodose reference on the skin back to 90% (Boutin et al. 1983).

We studied this approach in a randomized trial of 40 mesothelioma patients: 20 received radiotherapy, 20 did not. None of the 20 who received radiation developed malignant outgrowths from the chest wall; of the 20 who were not irradiated, 9 (45%, $p < 0.05$) developed nodules either along the thoracoscopy tract or along a thoracentesis tract. Since then, we have used preventive radiotherapy routinely in patients with mesothelioma and have no longer observed this problem.

We omit preventive radiotherapy in cases of metastatic pleural carcinomas since with these processes, chest wall seeding is not often seen.

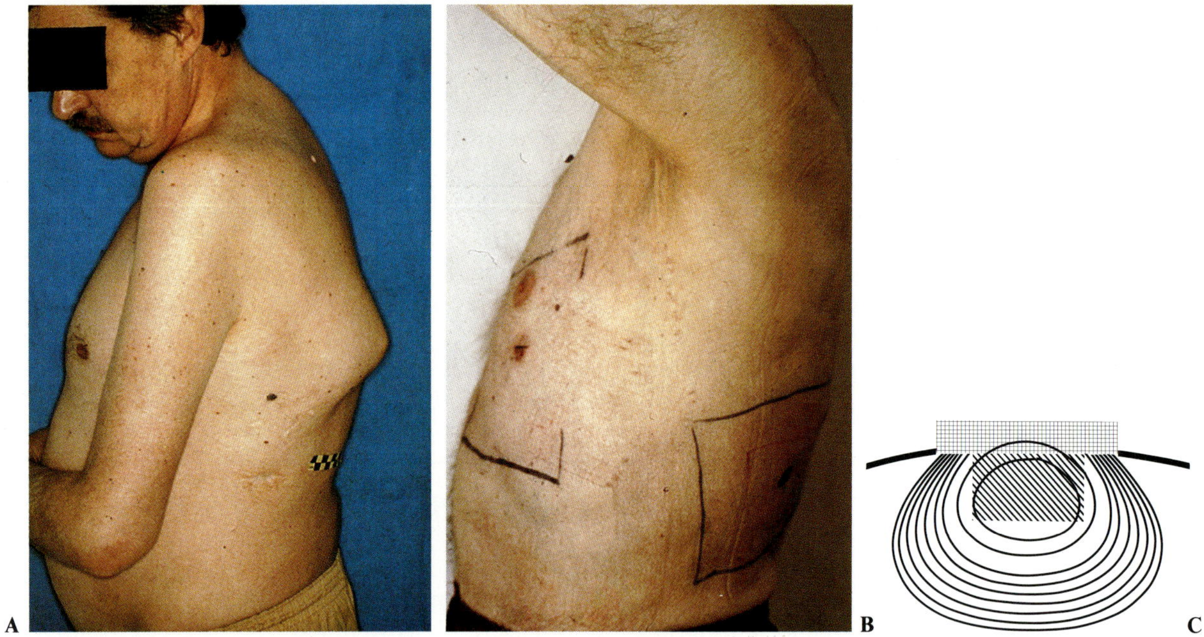

Fig. 34 A–C. Preventive radiotherapy in cases of mesothelioma. **A** This patient did not receive preventive radiotherapy. A large parietal tumor invasion developed on the needle track after a simple thoracentesis. The scar left by the thoracoscopy has not been invaded. **B** Areas receiving irradiation: the thoracoscopy scar on the chest wall and the needle puncture tracts on the back. **C** Diagram of radiation showing isodose curves: the 90% isodose curve is brought to the skin using a paraffin plaque. It is 3 cm deep

4.3 Pleural Drainage Technique (Table 1)

Drainage must be carried out quickly and completely. It is therefore best to use large bore chest tubes, between 24 and 32 Fr. Drainage can cause local discomfort due to the tube pressing on the soft tissue of the chest wall, which generally responds to simple oral analgesics such as paracetamol (acetaminophen), amidopyrine, etc., administered to the patient as needed.

4.3.1 Chest Tube Drainage of Short Duration

In simple diagnostic thoracoscopy for pleural effusion, all the fluid is removed before and during the procedure. The chest tube is therefore inserted to drain residual air from the thorax, allowing the lung to reexpand immediately to the chest wall. The tube is passed through the main point of entry and pushed posteriorly as close to the apex as possible. In most cases, total resolution of the pneumothorax occurs within minutes, as indicated by the cessation of bubbling through the water seal. The state of lung reexpansion is confirmed radiographically and the chest tube is removed while the patient is still on the thoracoscopy table. This makes for a very short period of discomfort for the patient, who is, therefore, generally not hesitant to repeat the examination at a later date if the effusion becomes chronic and requires pleurodesis. The patient can leave the hospital the following day after spending no more than 24–36 h away from home.

If pleural drainage requires more than 24 h, a Heimlich valve (Heimlich 1983) may be used in place of the water seal, allowing the patient to move about freely during the day.

4.3.2 Chest Tube Drainage of Medium Duration

After pulmonary biopsy. If the pulmonary breach is closed using electrocautery or laser (or closes spontaneously), the lung quickly returns to its normal position against the chest wall, and bubbling through the water seal ceases. In these

Table 1. Pleural Drainage

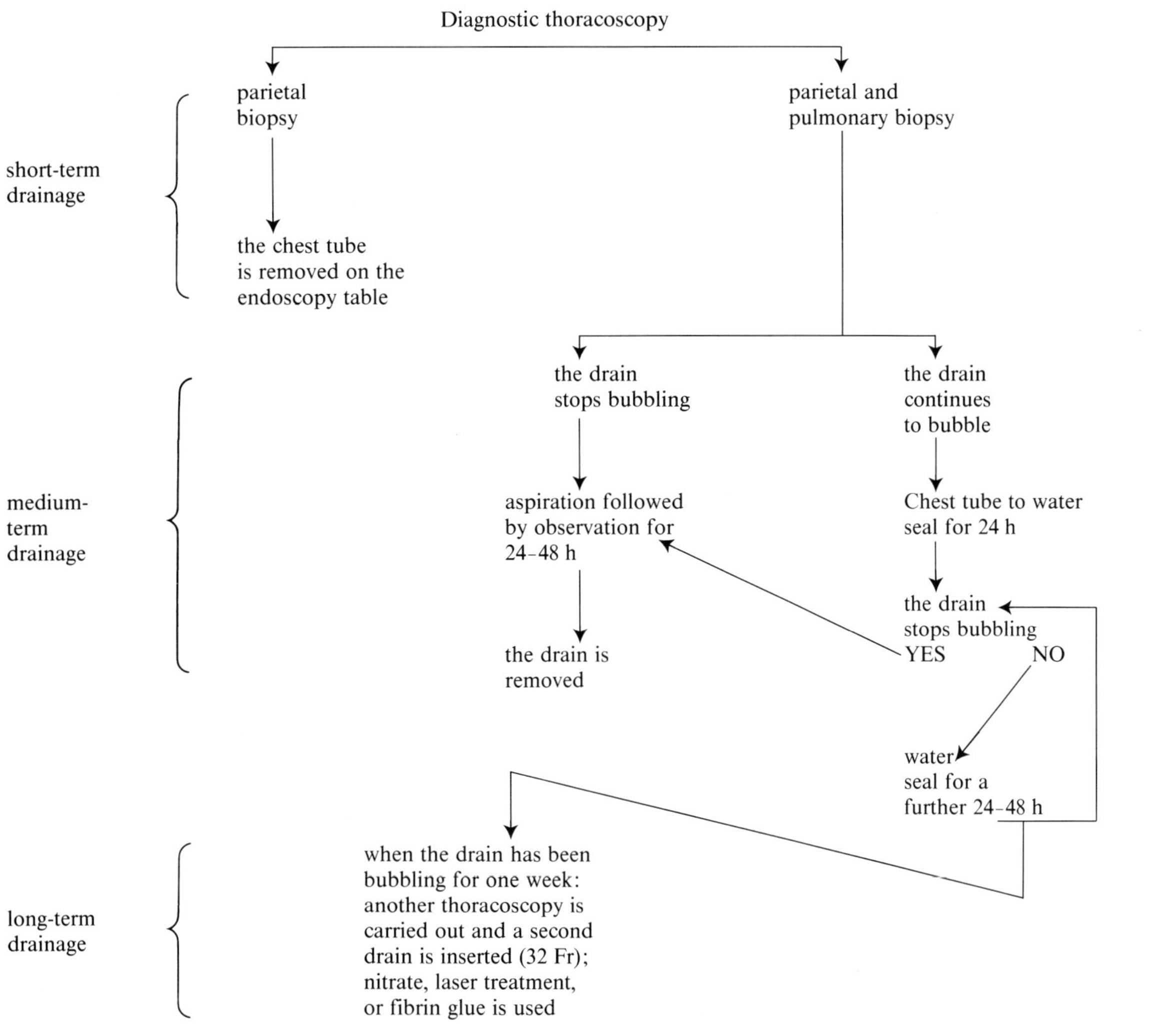

If drainage lasts more than 24 hours, a Heimlich valve is attached to the chest tube, enabling the patient to move about during the day. The patient undergoes physical therapy from the first day including exercises of the diaphragm and ribs

cases, apply -30 cm suction to the chest tube, which may be removed at 24–48 h without a clamping trial, if roentgenograms confirm that the lung is completely expanded.

If the chest tube continues to bubble through the water seal at the completion of the procedure, there is a persistent breach of the visceral pleura. Water-seal drainage is then continued until all bubbling stops, usually within 24 h. Then suction is applied as described above.

In our unit, chest tube drainage is continued an average of 2.6 ± 0.4 days after pulmonary biopsy.

Drainage after pleurodesis. The lung must be brought back against the chest wall as quickly as possible to minimize the possibility of adhesions forming in the still-contracted lung. A 28 or 30 Fr chest tube is sometimes positioned through a special point of entry, made under thoracoscopic control, on the lowest point of the mid- or posterior axillary line. The tube is pushed toward the apex posteriorly. We usually apply -30 to -50 cm H_2O suction to the tube on the first day and -50 to -100 cm H_2O from the second day onwards. The chest tube is removed as soon as the amount of fluid drainage drops below 100 ml per day, or on the sixth day at the latest. Indeed, the drain might leave, after 6 or 7 days, a track which will not heal easily, risking a cutaneous fistula. Drainage of more than 100 ml/day after 6 days is also proof that the attempt at pleurodesis has failed; it is thus pointless to continue drainage.

In our department, the average drainage times are: (a) 4.8 ± 0.4 days with talc poudrage for spontaneous pneumothorax, (b) 4.8 ± 0.2 days with talc poudrage for malignant effusion, (c) 5.6 ± 0.5 days with tetracycline instillation for malignant effusion, and (d) 5.8 ± 0.7 days with talc poudrage for transudative pleural effusions.

4.3.3 Long-Term Drainage (> 7 days)

This is rarely necessary but occurs in three situations: (a) chronic spontaneous pneumothorax where thoracotomy to oversew the defect is contraindicated due to the presence of cardiac and/or pulmonary failure; (b) empyema with broncho-pleural fistula; (c) prolonged air leak after pulmonary biopsy: persistent bubbling occurred three times in our series of 300 patients (1%).

Whenever the water seal continues to bubble, we leave the chest tube water sealed but omit suction, since it may keep the breach open. In such cases, we remove all suction devices from the bedside since it is a great temptation to turn on the suction to test for air leak (and this repeated testing may perpetuate the breach).

In all these cases the lung is to some extent nonadherent to the chest wall. If the lung is close to the chest wall, with the mediastinum in its normal, midline position, and there is no subcutaneous emphysema, there is no risk involved. The patient, though impatient to have his chest tube removed, is simply kept under observation. Eventually, the lung reexpands and reestablishes full contact with the chest wall; the drainage tube may then be removed after another 48 h. This entire process may take 8–14 days.

If the lung remains away from the chest wall and bubbling occurs with each exhalation, the flow from the fistula may well be greater than that of the drainage tube. As mentioned above, chest-tube suction must be avoided. The problem most often will be resolved if a second drainage tube is placed under direct vision by the thoracoscopist, using local anesthesia. This tube must also be of large bore (32 Fr) and is connected to a second water seal. It is most unusual for the flow from a bronchopleural fistula in a spontaneously breathing patient to be greater than that of two large-bore chest tubes.

We have carried out several consecutive thoracoscopies in patients with persistent fistulae, for diverse indications: in order to change the position of a drainage tube; to try to clean the edges of a pulmonary breach, to clean out a purulent pleural cavity; to use nitrate on the breach or refreshen its edges with a laser; or to try closure with biological adhesives. The problem here lies not only on the fistula itself, but relates to its cause (usually a malignant lesion), to a lack of pulmonary elasticity associated with deformed parenchyma or trapped lung, to the poor general state of the patient, to microbial resistance to antibiotics, etc. For these reasons, some patients with bronchopleural fistula may die in spite of extraordinary medical or surgical efforts.

4.4 Temperature Curve After Thoracoscopy (Fig. 35)

The average temperature curve is roughly normal. In 10%–20% of patients a slight fever as high as 38° C to 38.5° C may be measured, which

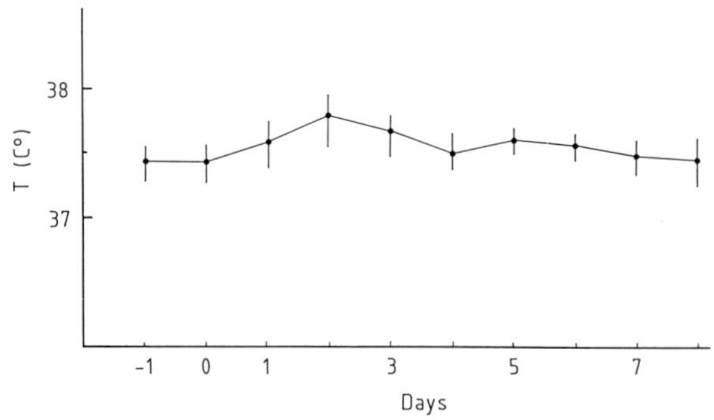

Fig. 35. Temperature curve after thoracoscopy. Mean curve of 300 thoracoscopies. There is almost no change in the patient mean temperature after thoracoscopy. This is especially true when the chest tube is removed within minutes to a few hours after the procedure

disappears either spontaneously or with anti-pyretic treatment within 24–36 h.

Some 2% of patients develop a mild bronchitis, perhaps related to bronchial obstruction or collapse during tube drainage, in spite of preventive measures instituted by physical therapists (incentive spirometry, breathing exercises, cough training, etc.). Prescription of B2-adrenergic aerosols with or without antibiotics for a few days will generally resolve this problem.

Finally, 2% of patients develop local infection at the wound site. This minor infection resolves quickly with local treatment and antibiotics.

In conclusion, it can be affirmed that thoracoscopy is a safe, high-yield procedure. The physician must take a certain number of precautions, but the rules are simple and relate largely to common sense. Aseptic conditions must be maintained, as for any pleural drainage, and the rare infectious complications that occur must be promptly identified and treated. Post-thoracoscopic observation is the same as that for any pleural drainage procedure, generally requiring 2 to 4 days and sometimes much less. The well-trained thoracoscopist will find the procedure easy to perform, well-tolerated by the patient, and with diagnostic and therapeutic results that easily justify the time spent in his training.

Chapter 5: Diagnostic Thoracoscopy for Pleural Effusions

5.1 Indications

The diagnosis of pleural effusions is the most important and the oldest indication for thoracoscopy, as described by Jacobaeus himself in his earliest articles. Many unselected pleural effusions defy even the most sophisticated investigators, despite comprehensive nonsurgical evaluation. A complete work-up includes the following (Light 1983, 1985; Sahn 1988): one or more thorough analyses of pleural fluid: biochemical, bacteriological, cytological and immunological (Rossi et al.1987); one or two pleural biopsy attempts using a biopsy needle (Abrams, Vim-Silverman, or Cope); microbiological and cytological sputum analysis; intradermal testing using tuberculin, as well as fungal antigens in endemic areas; bronchoscopy; and a thorough clinical and radiological assessment. Despite these tests and others which focus on the specifics of the patient being evaluated, approximately 20% of pleural effusions are still idiopathic after several weeks of observation.

Thoracoscopy is indicated in this 20% group of pleural exudates. Tuberculosis is sometimes suspected, but in recent decades malignancy has been found more frequently. Obviously, it is very important to proceed with further studies until a diagnosis is made or until the benefits of knowing the cause no longer warrant the morbidity of further investigation. We have reported a series of 1000 effusions which were followed for four or more weeks (Boutin et al. 1981a): the usual intensive studies failed to find the etiology in 215 patients. Thoracoscopy was carried out and showed 131 of the total 150 malignancies not yet diagnosed; thus only 4% remained "idiopathic" after thoracoscopy.

Waiting can be detrimental to the patient. In cases of malignant disease, diagnosis will, of course, become evident at some point, but delay in diagnosis makes therapeutic pleurodesis less likely to be effective: indeed, invasion of the visceral pleura by malignancy will result in a "trapped lung," causing an irreversible functional deficit.

Moreover, if efficient treatments to pleural cancer are to be discovered in the near future, they will have to be used as soon as possible, meaning that early diagnosis will require early thoracoscopy.

In cases of undiagnosed primary pleural tuberculosis, the specific histopathologic characteristics of tuberculous granulomas may spontaneously disappear after 3–4 weeks, making a definite diagnosis impossible (Boutin et al. 1968, 1975a).

In cases of idiopathic pleurisy, cancer can be largely eliminated as a potential etiology by performing extensive biopsies in the pleural cavity (Miller and Hatcher 1978). This negative information may be very reassuring to the patient. Furthermore, once infectious processes are ruled out, the clinician may consider a trial of corticosteroid therapy that might prevent further recurrence of the effusion and reduce eventual pleural scarring.

If diagnostic thoracoscopy is performed (Loddenkemper et al. 1978a, 1978b, 1981; Martenson et al. 1985, 1989), the sensitivity of diagnosis reaches 93%–97% in tuberculosis and cancer (Boutin et al. 1985a), based on biopsies and sometimes brushings of the pleural surface. Hormone-receptor assays on biopsy material provide further important information in cases of cancer of the breast or ovary (Levine et al. 1986). This diagnostic thoracoscopic procedure provides the lowest morbidity and inconvenience to the patient, since chest tube drainage is required for only 15–30 min until the lung reexpands to the chest wall. Thus, a very brief period of hospitalization is necessary, as previously discussed.

5.2 Metastatic Pleural Malignancies

Closed pleural needle biopsies (Huguenin-Dumittan and Dottrens 1981) are only successful at best in 50% of metastatic pleural malignancies (Fentiman et al. 1981; Chretien and Andre-Bougaran 1967; Mestitz et al. 1958; Migueres et al. 1974, 1975a; Sison and Weiss 1962). They are of little value with still-localized tumors (where thoracoscopy is already highly sensitive). They are of no use at all in metastatic tumors confined to the diaphragmatic, visceral, or mediastinal pleura (Canto et al. 1985b). On the other hand, the more the tumor is widespread within the parietal pleura, the more closed biopsy is likely to be positive. Thus, centers which see more advanced disease have a higher yield with closed pleural biopsy alone.

Similarly, variable results are obtained from the cytology of pleural fluid (Collins and Sahn 1987; Johnston 1985; Palojoki 1981; Renault 1978). In 95 cases of pleurisy, Salyer et al. (1975) obtained 53 positive needle biopsy results and 69 positive cytologies, the combination of the two methods giving a positive yield in 86 patients (90%). This high yield is achieved only in the advanced stages of disease. A yield of 50%–60% from pleural fluid cytology is certainly a more representative figure (Dines et al., 1975). Graham et al. (1953) studied 338 patients with negative cytology in 221 cases, of which 114 eventually were proved to have malignant pleural disease (48% false negative).

The importance of thoracoscopy certainly is in making an early diagnosis when the two conventional methods of pleural biopsy and pleural fluid cytology have failed (Boutin et al. 1980; Lagèze et al. 1960; Weissberg et al. 1980a; Wihlm et al. 1981).

The endoscopic appearance (Figs. 36–39) is suggestive of malignancy in over 86% of cases (Table 2), and discloses the following aspects:

1. *Nodules* which are 1 to 5 mm in diameter
2. *Polypoid lesions* of somewhat larger dimensions
3. Still larger localized tumoral *masses*
4. Malignant *thickening* of the pleura, whitish, with an irregular, pebbly surface; pachypleuritis is hard, with little vascularity
5. Localized white "candle wax drops."

One should not be satisfied, however, with the macroscopic appearance, which can be misleading. Some malignancies look like nonspecific inflammation and, conversely, certain inflammatory lesions can look like tumors (see Fig. 50). Even mesotheliomas, which often have a fairly characteristic grape-like nodular form, can look like ordinary inflammation. Endoscopic appearance,

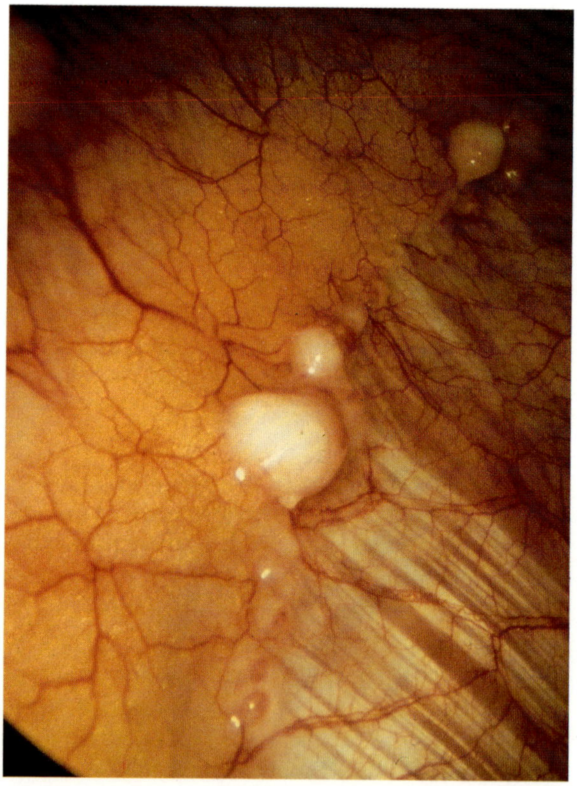

Fig. 36. Secondary cancers: Metastases in the intercostal space. The rib is covered with a fatty yellow plaque. The internal intercostal muscle fibers are clearly visible. There are metastatic nodules all along the lymphatic vessels running through the intercostal space. An Abrams biopsy is unlikely to be successful in sampling such localized processes

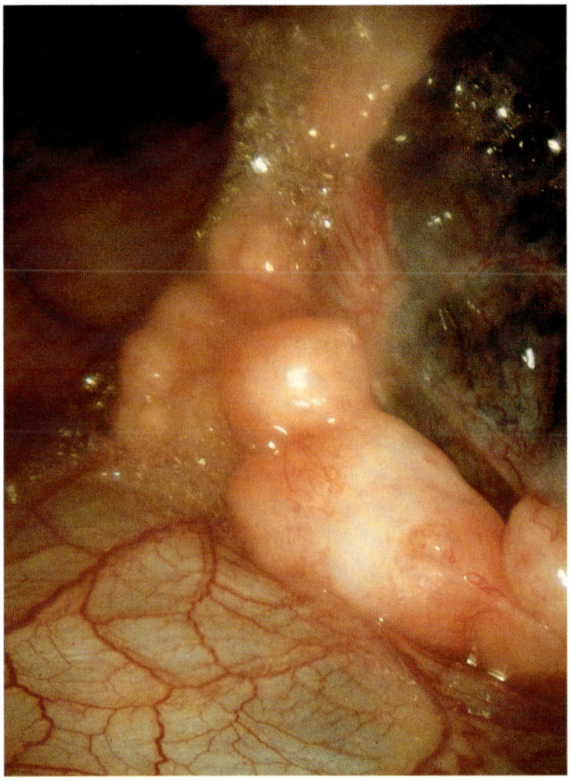

Fig. 37. Secondary cancers: pulmonary and diaphragmatic metastases. Malignant nodules: the diaphragm, which is normal, can be seen at the *bottom*. The lung is on the *right*, and has brownish patches of anthracotic pigment. It is attached to the diaphragm and covered with white metastases. These lesions are inaccessible to closed pleural needle biopsy techniques. (Abrams, Cope, etc.)

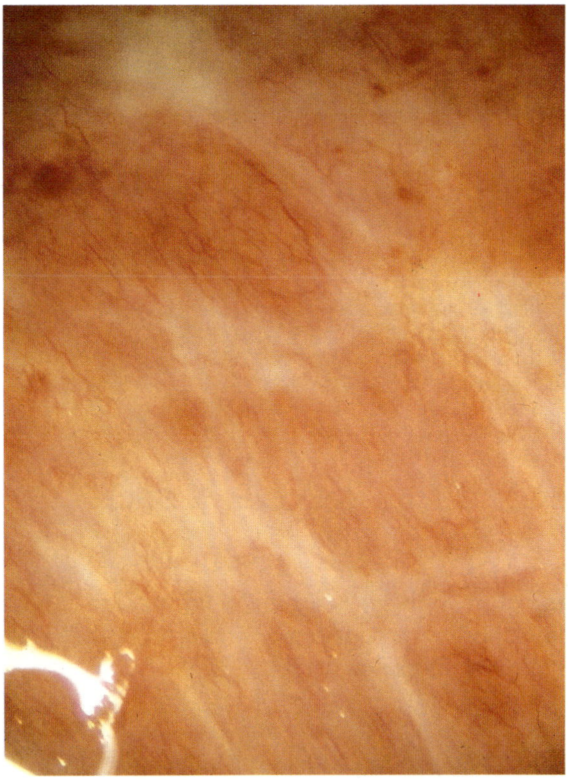

Fig. 39. Malignant lymphangitis. An irregular, white "network" can be seen; in some places it gets thicker, resembling candle wax droppings. When biopsied, the lesions cut cleanly and do not hemorrhage. This was a case of invasion of the pleura by chronic lymphoid leukemia. At an early stage of mesothelioma, such an aspect of lymphangitis may be observed. The photo was taken using high magnification; each lymphatic vessel has a diameter of 0.5–1 mm

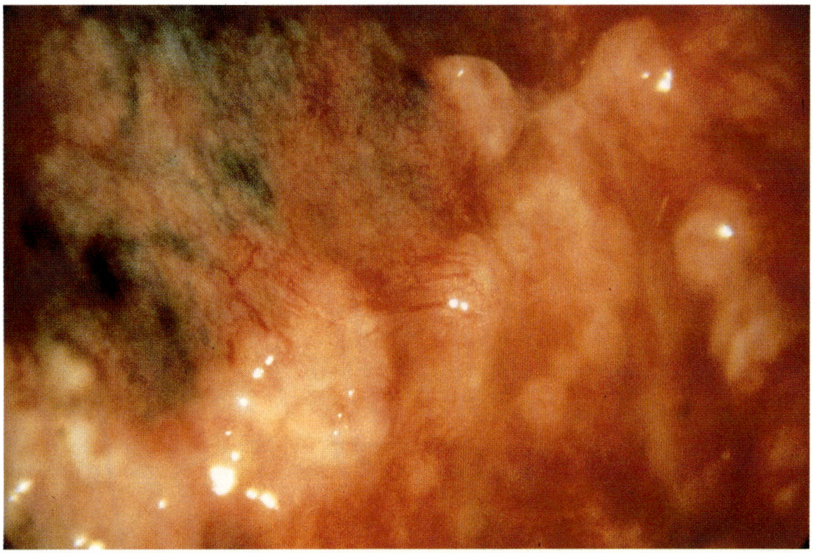

Fig. 38. Metastases on the visceral pleura. The lung is covered with numerous metastatic nodules which are easy to biopsy. Only part of the lung on the *top left* is normal

Table 2. Endoscopic appearance of pleural malignancies in 200 patients. Endoscopically there is no significant difference in appearance between cases of metastatic cancer and mesothelioma, except for the "grape-like" appearance which occurs mainly in cases of mesothelioma. Because of the possibility of nonspecific findings in malignant diseases, large numbers of biopsies must be taken in suspicious cases

	Metastasis	Mesothelioma	*P*
Patients *(n)*	100	100	
1. Nodules-masses	40	35	NS
2. Pleural thickening	30	20	NS
3. Combinations of the above (1+2)	10	12	NS
4. "Grape-like" appearance	3	23	<0,01
5. Lymphangitis	6	2	NS
6. Nonspecific abnormalities	11	8	NS

therefore, only gives a general impression, which must always be confirmed by microscopic examination of biopsy material.

5.2.1 Topography of Pleural Malignancies

The topography of pleural malignancies was studied by Canto et al. (1983) (Fig. 40). In 94% of their cases the lower half of the pleural cavity was affected, which justifies a low point of entry, either the sixth or seventh intercostal space. In 28% of cases, only the visceral pleura was involved, hence closed needle biopsy could not succeed. In breast cancer, lesions frequently occur on the anterior ipsilateral parietal pleura.

5.2.2 Histopathological Results

Histopathological results are the only criteria for certain diagnoses. In our series the sensitivity of biopsy increased with the years, rising from 78% early in our experience to 97% after we had perfected the thoracoscopic equipment and gained greater experience (Boutin et al. 1985a).

We have reviewed (Boutin et al. 1981d) 4301 reported cases of diagnostic thoracoscopy using rigid instruments in cases of chronic pleural effusion from 21 different studies. Of 1472 cancer cases, 1333 correct pathologic diagnoses (92.5%) were achieved from thoracoscopic specimens. *But why are 7.5% of thoracoscopic biopsies negative?* Several answers have been advanced:

1. In some patients with cancer, pleural effusion is due not to malignant pleural invasion but to malignant obstruction of mediastinal or pul-

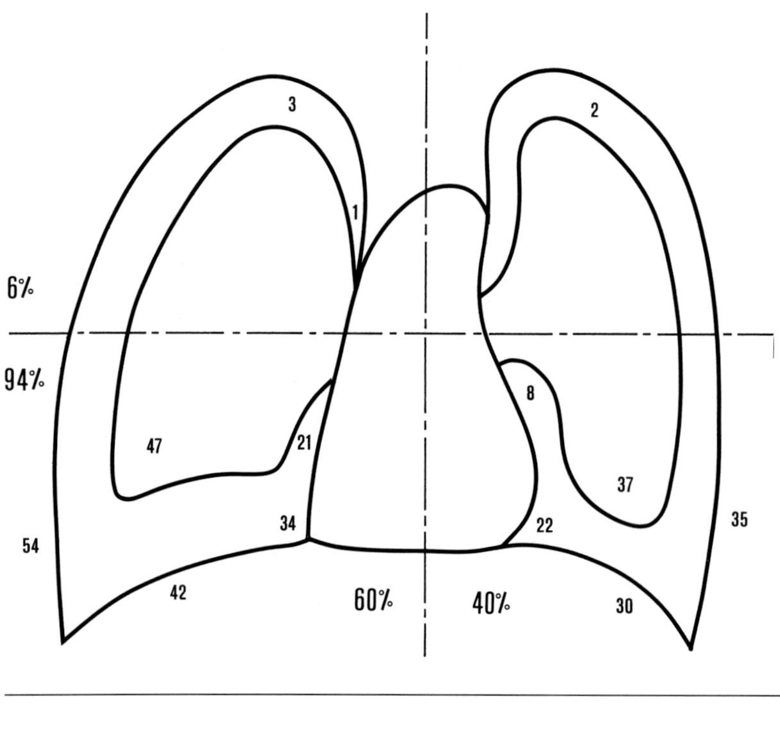

Fig. 40. Location of cancers in the pleural cavity. In 183 cases of primary or secondary cancer of the pleura, there was a predominance of lesions in the inferior half of the pleural cavity; note the prevalence of tumors invading the diaphragm, the visceral pleura, the mediastinum, and the pericardium, none of which can be biopsied using Abrams or Cope needle (From Canto et al. 1981, 1983, 1989)

monary lymphatics, which are not biopsied. This has been described both in lung cancer (Brinkman 1959; Decker et al. 1978; Tandon 1966) and cancer of the breast (Weichselbaum et al. 1977).
2. Rarely, an effusion is the late consequence of lymphatic obstruction due to mediastinal radiotherapy (Whitcomb and Schwartz 1971), which occurred in 1% of cases in our series.
3. The thoracoscopist learns with experience and has a suboptimal yield initially.
4. Multiple biopsies must be taken systematically. There is no such thing as "too many." The costovertebral gutter and the diaphragm must be routinely sampled. Remember that metastases can sometimes not be recognized endoscopically (Morino et al. 1977).
5. If the biopsy is reported as negative in suspected malignancy, the pathologist should be asked to section all tissue, including "deepers" and to completely review all slides. This has enabled us to obtain additional diagnoses in several cases.
6. Sometimes the pleura is covered with a fibrinous, necrotic layer which requires removal in order to biopsy the parietal pleura behind it.
7. But the major stumbling block of thoracoscopy lies in cases of adherent pleura! Once again the experience of the physician is paramount in being able to biopsy after dividing and cutting adhesions. There are, however, cases where this is impossible. In our routine experience, where we have managed to achieve 97% sensitivity in cancerous effusions, false negative findings were universally due to adhesions which denied access to the neoplastic tissue.

5.2.3 Cancer of the Lung

Although pleural effusion with lung cancer usually indicates nonresectibility due to tumor invasion of the pleura or mediastinum, some cases have been resected and cured. Indeed, the Mayo Clinic group (Decker et al. 1978) found four patients with negative cytologies whose pleural effusions were due to obstructive atelectasis or infection. These four patients had pulmonary resection and survived more than five years free of disease. In the view of some investigators, thoracoscopy is the ideal technique for staging of these cancer patients. Weissberg et al. (1981c) performed thoracoscopies in 45 patients with lung cancer and pleural effusion. In 37 they found pleural invasion; three patients had mediastinal disease; the remaining five patients had no evident metastatic disease and, therefore, no contraindication to resection. Canto et al. (1985b) found similar results; eight of 44 patients (18%) had no thoracoscopic evidence of pleural disease and six actually went to resection. Thus, it would appear that some cases with negative pleural biopsy and pleural fluid cytology deserve a staging thoracoscopy before ruling out thoracotomy and surgical resection.

5.2.4 Breast Cancer and Other Hormone-Dependent Cancers

With metastatic pleural effusion, thoracoscopy provides a relatively simple way to collect tissue for hormone-receptor assay, which helps in the selection of effective treatment for breast cancer and other hormone-dependent cancers. This is particularly so in patients whose primary cancer was removed before this assay was generally available (Levine et al. 1986).

5.3 Diffuse Malignant Mesothelioma

Mesothelioma is one of the best indications for thoracoscopy; it is much less invasive than thoracotomy and allows equally good tissue sampling for pathological diagnosis (Boutin et al. 1988a, 1986c, 1989b; Martenson, 1981; Martenson et al. 1984).

5.3.1 Indications for Thoracoscopy

Thoracoscopy is indicated in practically all cases of suspected mesothelioma. In our series of 157 patients (Boutin et al. 1989d), the indications were as follows: 88% patients had chronic pleurisy; 2% had empyema, 1% had a chronic spon-

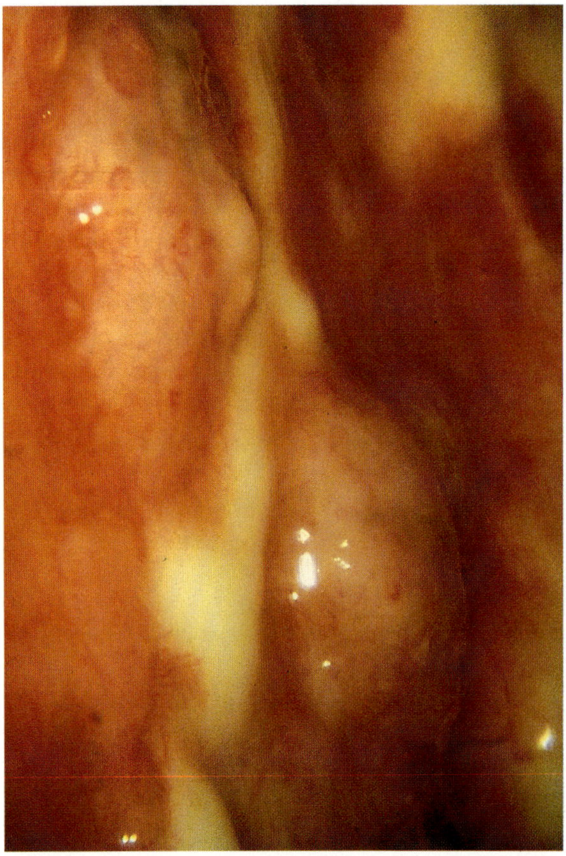

Fig. 41. Mesothelioma - stage I. In this patient, formerly an asbestos worker, yellowish, fibrohyalin parietal plaques can be seen. Malignant nodules protrude between these plaques. This aspect is quite characteristic, but relatively rare: firstly, because mesothelioma often occurs in patients who have no pleural plaques (68% of cases in our series); secondly, the nodules were limited to the posterior parts of the parietal pleura and the diaphragm; and neither the lung nor the mediastinum were affected (stage IA). These limited nodules with a diameter of 3-4 mm are easier to see with the thoracoscope than on CT scan

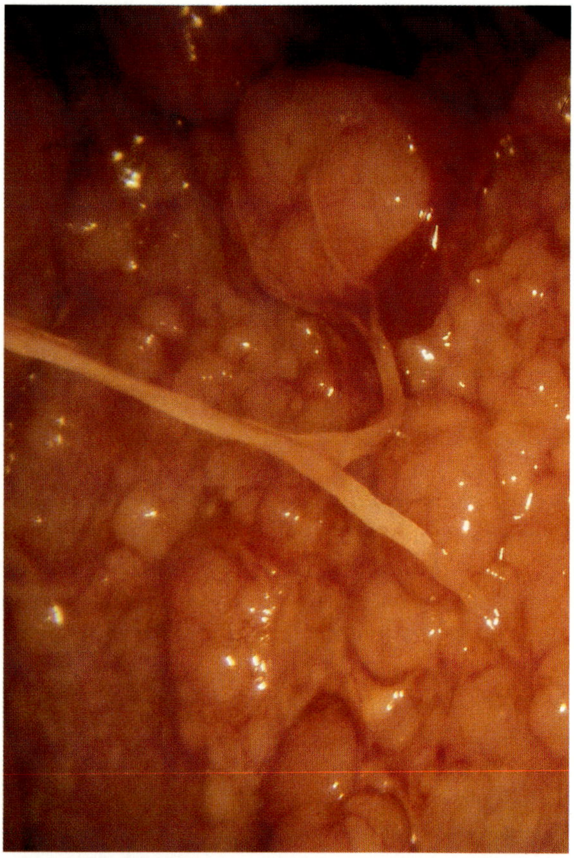

Fig. 42. Mesothelioma - stage II. The widespread appearance of mesothelioma is clearly seen here. The parietal pleura, as well as visceral and mediastinal pleura, have been completely invaded by a thick, malignant pachypleuritis. Several nodules of different sizes stand out against this background. The largest, on the *top*, is 10-12 mm in diameter; the others are 3-5 mm in diameter. When biopsied, they proved to have a very hard consistency

taneous pneumothorax, and 9% presented with pleural nodules without effusion on roentgenograms. Of these patients, 80% recalled previous exposure to asbestos.

5.3.2 Macroscopic Examination

In our 157 patients, the pleural cavity was usually free of adhesions or presented only localized fibrinous attachments, which did not obstruct examination. In 30 patients, however, there were adhesions significant enough to require lysis with laser or electrocoagulation. In only nine patients were there such extensive adhesions that an adequate exploration of the pleura was impossible: these nine were referred to surgery for diagnostic thoracotomy. In the majority of our cases the tumor presented endoscopically as nodules or masses ranging from several millimeters (Fig. 41) to 5-10 cm in diameter. In most patients the nodules and masses were associated with a more general thickening of the pleura of several millimeters (Fig. 42). In 10% of the cases the nodules were small, between 1 and 5 mm in diameter; the other 90% had larger nodules spread over the

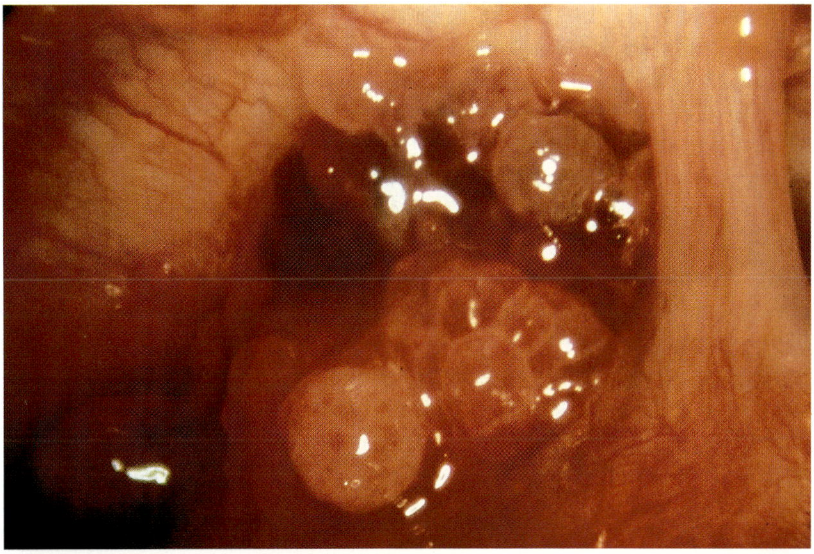

Fig. 43. Mesothelioma: nodules with "grape-like" appearance. On the right, at the base of a pleuro-pulmonary adhesion, there are nodules which are typically shiny and have the appearance of a grape; a thick, viscous liquid escapes when biopsies are taken. This is common in cases of mesothelioma and could be said to be characteristic although the same occurs occasionally in some cases of metastatic disease (especially of the ovary)

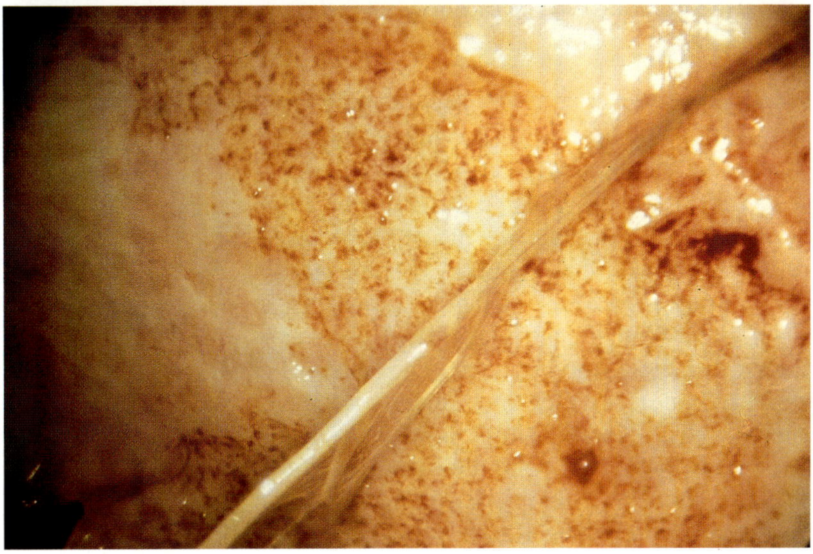

Fig. 44. Mesothelioma: parietal lymphangitis associated with fibrohyaline pleural plaques. A fibrinous adhesion runs diagonally across the *foreground* of the photo. There are white, asbestotic, fibrohyalin pleural plaques on the *top right* and the *left*. Diffuse parietal malignant lymphangitis can be seen between these plaques. There is a progression from the photo in Fig. 39, where the lymphatic network is slack, to this photo where it is much tighter

surface of the parietal or diaphragmatic pleura. Typically, these nodules are clear to yellowish white, with little vascularity, translucent, smooth, sessile or polypoid, sometimes having a grape-like appearance (Fig. 43). This is a characteristic of mesotheliomas, but not confined to them, as we also found it in 3% of cases of metastatic cancer of the pleura (Table 2). When biopsied, they are sometimes friable and filled with viscous fluid, or hard and difficult to biopsy.

A malignant thickening of the pleura, usually 2–5 mm thick, is hard, with little elasticity, as opposed to benign inflammatory pachypleuritis. When biopsied the section cuts cleanly in one piece, and there is no bleeding.

In 10% of our mesotheliomas, the lesions observed during thoracoscopy did not present any specific macroscopic characteristics: they appear as innocuous-looking inflammation of the pleural surface, occasionally with lymphangitis (Figs. 39, 44). In these cases, numerous biopsies must be carried out to yield a positive diagnosis.

An important step in staging mesotheliomas is to assess the extent of disease to the visceral pleura and the lung, which can easily be seen during thoracoscopy. The visceral pleura always demonstrates less disease than the parietal pleura, especially in the early stages of the illness: there are fewer nodules, which are smaller in size. In fact, in 19 cases the visceral pleura appeared normal endoscopically, an impression we confirmed with systematic biopsies.

In four patients who underwent two thoracoscopies 6 months apart, we found that the nodules, initially quite small, appeared only on the parietal and diaphragmatic pleura at the beginning of the illness. At the time of the second procedure these nodules had grown to masses as large as 8–10 cm in diameter, and the mesothelioma had visibly invaded the formerly normal visceral pleura and lung.

5.3.3 Histopathological Aspects of Mesothelioma (Table 3)

The diagnostic accuracy of cytological study in mesothelioma is generally low, but widely variable in the literature from 0% to 64% (Brenner et al. 1982; Griffiths et al. 1980; Law et al. 1983; Matzel 1985; Ratzer et al. 1967; Taryle et al. 1976; Triol et al. 1984). Similarly, pleural needle biopsy produces a wide range of specificity, from 6% to 38%. Herbert and Gallagher (1982) concluded that the sensitivity of the two methods is poor and most investigators, therefore, prefer open surgical biopsy. The following indicates that thoracoscopy is a good alternative to thoracotomy: although two nondiagnostic examinations were reported by Ratzer et al. (1967) and only 13 of 23 were correctly diagnosed in a series by Law et al. (1984), fully 23 of 24 thoracoscopies were diagnostic in Martensson et al. series (1984), in which 17 mesotheliomas were distinguished from five carcinomas. Hirsch et al. (1982) reported nine out of nine correct diagnoses and Lewis et al. (1981) 28 out of 28. In our series, pathologic confirmation of the mesothelioma was obtained in every case where biopsies could be performed; that is, in 148 of 157 patients (94%) (Boutin et al. 1989 d): thoracotomy with surgical biopsy was, therefore, only required in nine patients. In our series, the Abram's needle sensitivity was 24% and that of fluid cytology was similar, 23%. These mesotheliomas were classified pathologically as 67% epithelial, 15% fibrosarcomatous, and 18% mixed cell.

Table 3. Diffuse, malignant mesothelioma: sensitivity of diagnostic techniques

	Patients	Positive results	
	(n)	*(n)*	(%)
Cytology of pleural fluid	152	35	23
Abrams biopsy	135	33	24
Thoracoscopy	157	148	94
Surgery (thoracotomy)	9	9	100

A positive result was achieved in every thoracoscopy where it was possible to take a biopsy, i.e. in 148 patients. Nine patients presented with tight symphysis which could not be separated; in these cases, the diagnosis was made by thoracotomy

To summarize, random closed pleural biopsies and pleural fluid cytology in mesotheliomas tend to lack specific features for the pathologist to be certain of the diagnosis, thus generally requiring directed biopsies through the thoracoscope or during thoracotomy. Both techniques have a similar diagnostic yield. However, we prefer thoracoscopy because of its far lower morbidity and pain.

5.3.4 Prognostic Aspects of Mesothelioma

Epithelial mesotheliomas, which are the most common, have a prognosis which is statistically better than fibrosarcomatous mesotheliomas: in our series, median survival rates were 383 days for epithelial types versus only 138 days for fibrosarcomatous types ($p < 0.02$).

Thoracoscopy enabled us to divide stage I as described by Butchart et al. (1976) and others (Antman 1980; Brenner et al. 1982; Chahinian 1983) into two subcategories (Fig. 45):

Stage IA (Fig. 41). The parietal and/or diaphragmatic pleura are involved, but the visceral pleura and mediastinum appear free of disease both thoracoscopically and on CT scan (19 patients in our series).

Stage IB (Figs. 46, 47) = Stage IA plus evident visceral pleural involvement but without invasion of the mediastinal pleura (70 patients).

The actuarial survival curves depending on stages are shown in Fig. 48 (Boutin et al. 1989 d). The median survival of stage IA patients is 27 months: patients undergoing surgery at this

Fig. 45. Stages of development of mesothelioma.

Stage I *A* Restricted to the parietal pleura or to the diaphragm
B Stage IA + ipsilateral visceral pleural invasion

Stage II Ipsilateral seeding (thoracic wall, mediastinum or pericardium) or controlateral seeding

Stage III Direct extension to the abdomen or to juxtathoracic lymph nodes

Stage IV Distant metastases

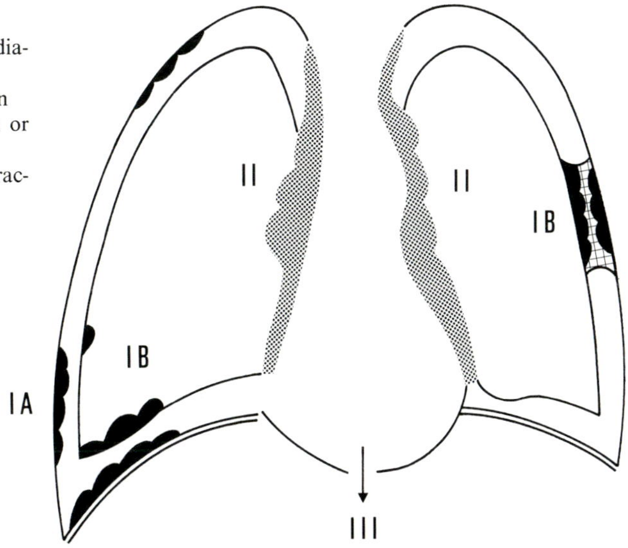

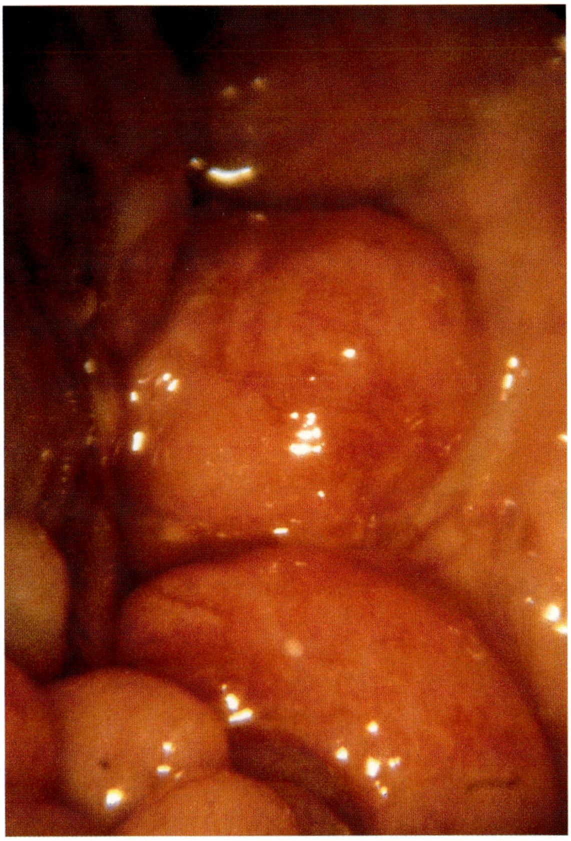

Fig. 46. Advanced stage of mesothelioma. Nodules are burgeoning all over the parietal pleura. This is the classic tumorous appearance of advanced mesothelioma. Large nodules have diameters of up to several centimeters

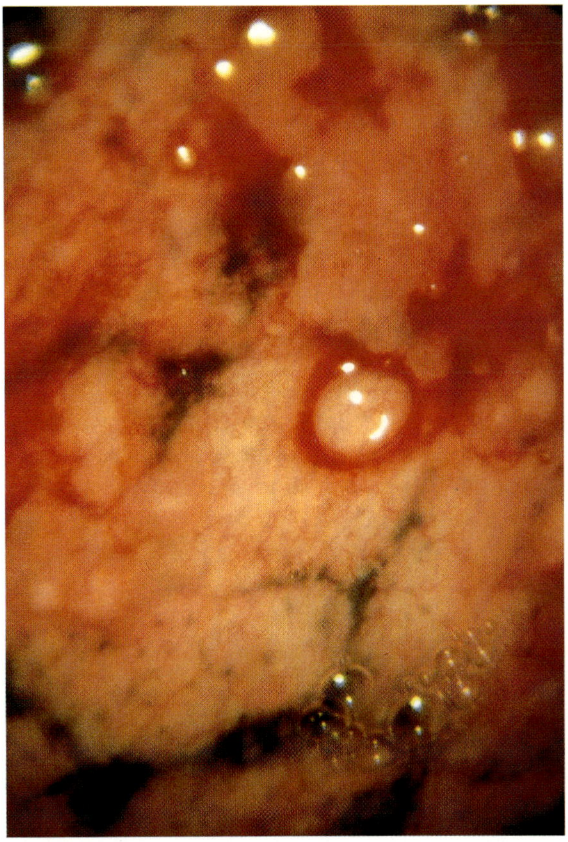

Fig. 47. Mesothelioma invading the visceral pleura. This photograph is from the same patient as on Fig. 46. Although his mesothelioma was in an advanced stage, it is clear to the naked eye that the visceral pleura and the lung have not been invaded to the same extent as the parietal pleura. The usual anthracotic pigment is still quite visible. The nodule in the *center* of the photo is 4 mm in diameter. Mesothelioma invades first the costal or diaphragmatic pleura, and later the visceral pleura and the lung

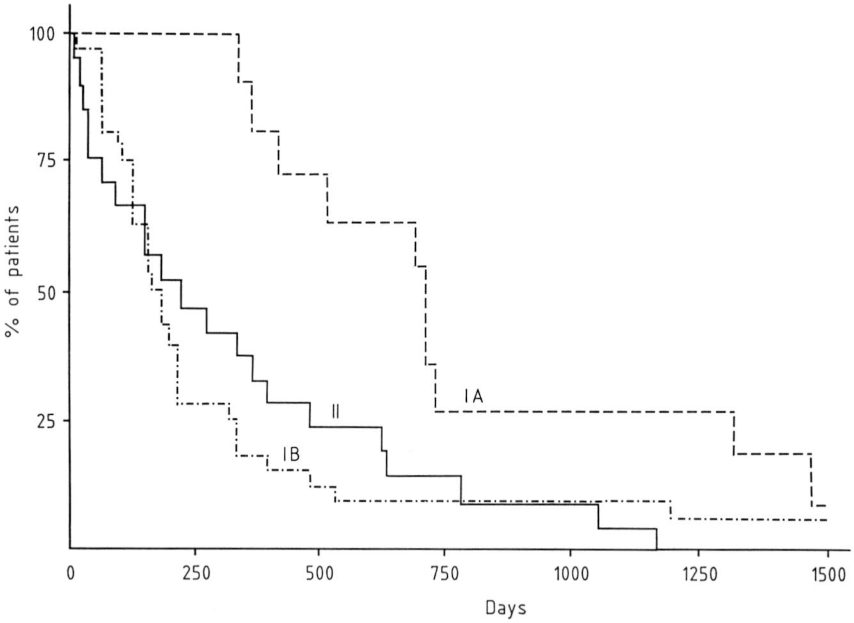

Fig. 48. Mesothelioma: actuarial survival curves. Actuarial survival (in days) according to staging. IA, 19 patients; IB, 70 patients; II, 72 patients. There is a significant difference between stage IA and stage IB survivals. By contrast, there is no statistical difference between stage IB and stage II survivals. The prognosis for stages III and IV is even worse

stage have an expected survival of 28.5 months compared to 26.5 months for those not operated. The value of surgery, therefore, appears to be entirely hypothetical, even at an early stage.

Median survival is only 11 months at stage IB. Thus, as soon as the visceral pleura is invaded, the prognosis becomes much worse, whatever treatment is attempted. In stage II, where the mediastinum is involved, survival is only 10 months, suggesting that mediastinal involvement may occur very soon after visceral pleural invasion.

5.4 Tuberculous Pleural Effusions (Figs. 49, 50)

Much less common at present, tuberculosis now causes less than 10% of all effusions seen in Europe and the USA, and a still lower percentage of all chronic cases. A diagnostic yield of 70%-90% may be achieved using an Abram's needle biopsy (Chrétien and André-Bougaran 1967; Boutin et al. 1968) for pathologic and cultural specimens, in conjunction with first morning gastric aspirates for tuberculosis culture. A second needle biopsy further enhances the yield, so that a definite diagnosis can be made in 95% of the cases. In our practice, therefore, thoracoscopy plays no significant role in this disease, and the discovery of tuberculous granulomata on thoracoscopic biopsy usually comes as a surprise.

Endoscopic appearance has been well described: grayish-white granulomata spread uniformly over the whole of the parietal and diaphragmatic pleura, with a clear concentration in the costovertebral gutter. There are many bands and adhesions, which can obstruct examination (Boutin et al. 1979). Lesions have often lost any specificity in their appearance by the time of thoracoscopy, however, resembling simple inflammatory change, with increased vascularity, a reddish color, an important and sometimes hemorrhagic fibrinous reaction, and numerous adhesions. These adhesions may limit the examiner and explain why the sensitivity of thoracoscopic biopsy is only 93% in our series. Even culture of biopsy fragments yields only 50% positive results, due probably to relatively low numbers of organisms in this form of tuberculosis, and to problems of sampling when faced with widespread adhesions.

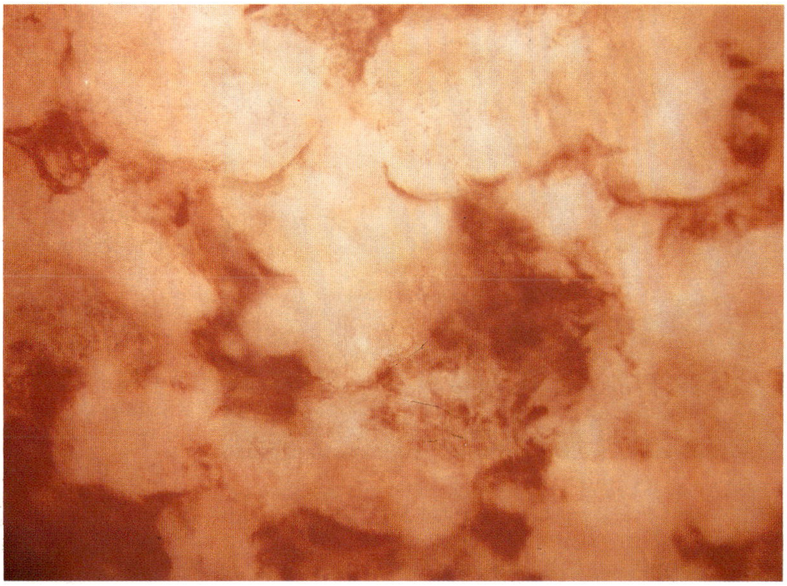

Fig. 49. Nodular, parietal tuberculosis. The parietal pleura is completely invaded by inflammatory rounded follicles which are confluent, with no healthy tissue between them. They are 2–4 mm in diameter. A diagnosis of tuberculosis is generally achieved in such cases by performing a needle biopsy. Thoracoscopy is thus only useful when a definite histopathologic or bacteriologic diagnosis cannot be obtained by usual procedures, i. e., mainly when pleurisy has become chronic

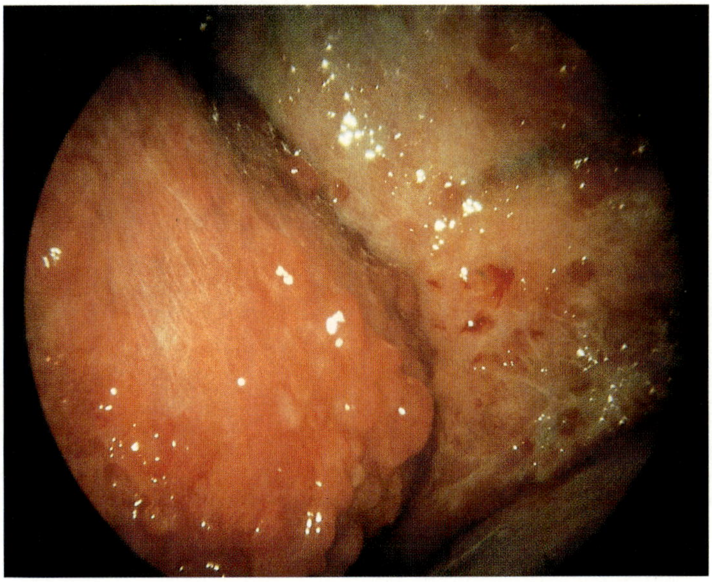

Fig. 50. Pleuropulmonary tuberculosis. In later stages, tuberculous lesions lose their characteristic appearance; the pleura is gradually invaded by more collagenous, fibroelastic tissue. This results in a white, soft appearance of the parietal pleura, resembling nonspecific inflammatory pachypleuritis, as can be seen on the *right* of the photo. In rarer cases the lung can be affected, as shown on the *left* of the photo; its surface resembles a tumor which must be ruled out by biopsy. In most cases of tuberculosis there are a large number of fibrinous adhesions, although this was not the case in this patient

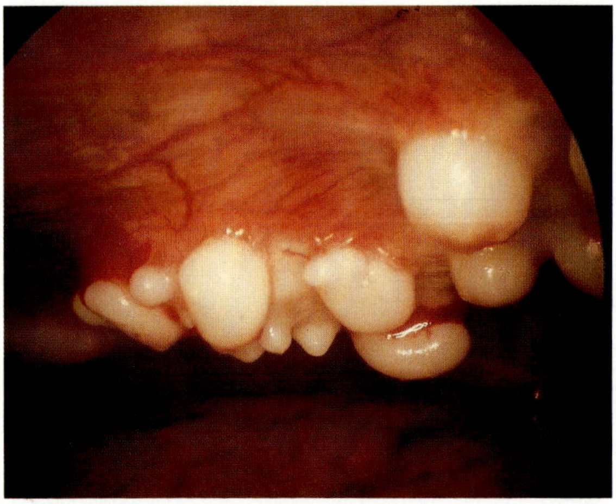

Fig. 51. Small round calcified asbestotic pleural plaques. Small, round pleural plaques resembling teeth or large pearls. On simple roentgenograms, these plaques are round and may suggest parenchymal neoplasms (pseudotumors). CT scan is sometimes useful in characterizing these lesions as pleural based, rather than parenchymal

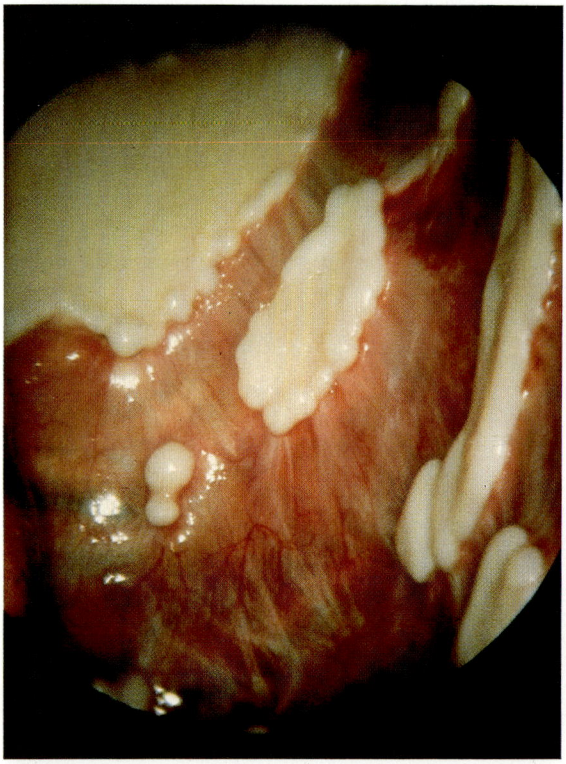

Fig. 52. Large calcified asbestotic pleural plaques. Asbestotic pleural plaques are scattered all over the parietal pleura. They are pearly white, with clear, shiny edges, and of a characteristically hard consistency. If the parietal plaques are not too large, they are usually found on the internal side of the ribs, not in the intercostal spaces, as in this photograph. However, when larger, they can form a "bridge" from one rib to the next

5.5 Miscellaneous Causes of Chronic Pleurisy

1. Asbestotic Pleurisy (Figs. 51, 52): Fibrohyaline or calcified pleural plaques, thick, pearly white, are found in asbestotic effusions. Thoracoscopic pulmonary biopsy may demonstrate high concentrations of asbestos fibers or fibrosis, providing further support to the diagnosis of industrial disease.
2. Rheumatoid Pleurisy: In nine cases of rheumatoid pleurisy, Faurschou (1974, 1985b, 1989) reported vesicles of 0.5 mm in diameter, translucent, resembling grains of sand, scattered over the parietal pleura.
3. Cardiac Effusion (Fig. 53): In this transudative process, endoscopic examination shows the pleura to be only slightly inflamed and whitish in color. The pleura is thickened due to edema, but transparent; the acinar outlines are prominent; vessels are suffused. There may be a plexus of lymphangitis on the visceral pleura. Adhesions arc uncommon.
4. Sarcoidosis (Fig. 54): A surfeit of grayish granulomata may be seen across the visceral surfaces, occasionally on the parietal pleura, all of which are easy to biopsy.
5. In all other cases of nonpurulent effusions, there is no specific macroscopic and microscopic appearance: the essential task is to eliminate malignant disease.

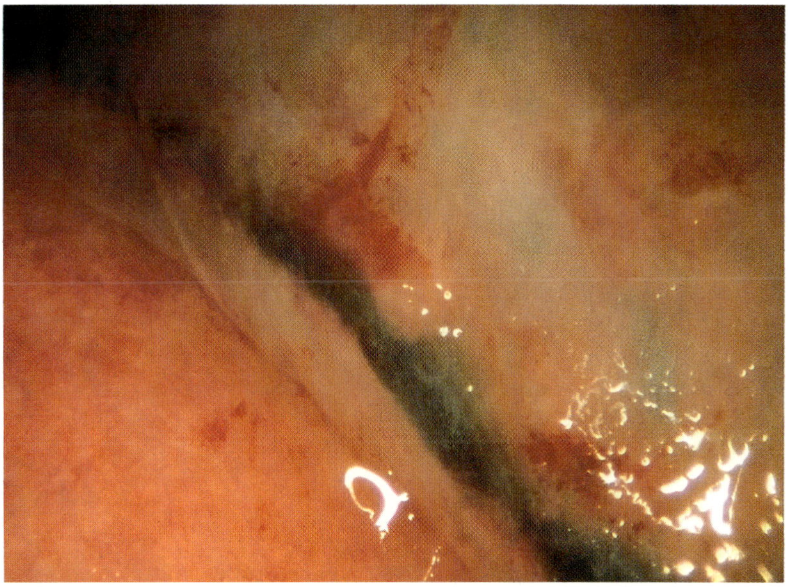

Fig. 53. Cardiac pleurisy. Left ventricular failure: a transudative effusion which has progressed to inflammatory in the chronic stage. The intercostal vein, in the *center* of the photo, is very dilated. On the *top right,* the pleura is edematous, white, opalescent and thick. On the *bottom left,* it is reddish and slightly inflammatory: simple mesothelial hyperplasia at biopsy

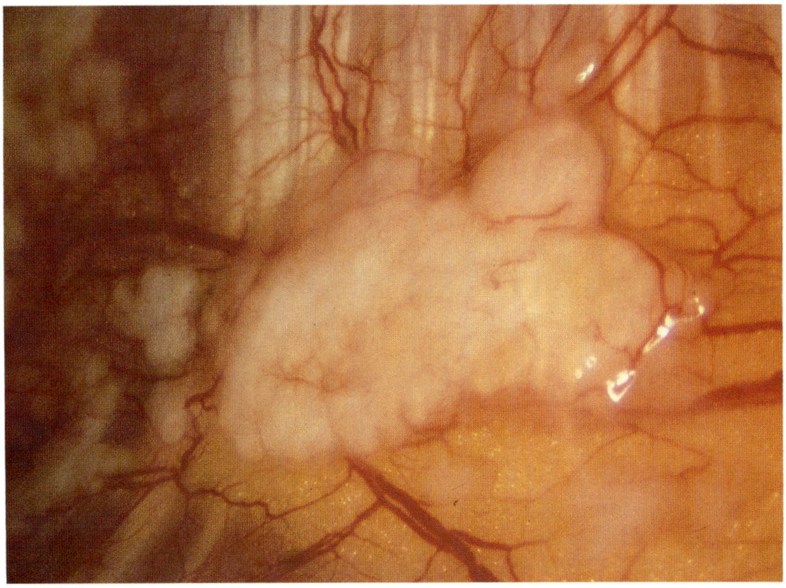

Fig. 54. Sarcoidosis. Pleural effusion in sarcoidosis is relatively uncommon. The parietal pleura is often affected by sarcoidosis. The same round, grey, opalescent granulations can be seen as on the visceral pleura. They are easy to biopsy. The granulomatous appearance resembles tuberculosis but without inflammation. There is no pachypleuritis, no congestion, no fibrin and there are no adhesions

Chapter 6: Pleurodesis for Chronic Pleural Effusion

The large number of recommended methods to obliterate the pleural space (pleurodesis), thereby preventing fluid reaccumulation, reflects the incompletely satisfactory results with any of the current techniques: existing practices each have advantages and disadvantages. Furthermore, publications on the subject are quite subject to fashion. Each new procedure brings with it a wave of glowing uncontrolled reports until another fad comes along and replaces it. It is therefore difficult to be very objective in choosing the best treatment for each type of patient (Hausheer and Yarbro 1985).

6.1 Which Types of Pleurisy Require Pleurodesis?

Predominantly malignant effusions require pleurodesis, which should not be recommended too hastily, however.

1. In chemotherapy- or hormone-sensitive tumors such as lymphomas and other hematological malignancies (Viallat et al. 1986a, 1986b), breast cancer, and ovarian cancer, a suitable systemic treatment should be tried first (Fentiman et al. 1983; Fentiman 1987; Migueres and Jover 1981).
2. The effusion must be disabling and the patient must get unequivocal subjective benefit, albeit temporary, from simple pleural puncture with fluid aspiration. It must be remembered that patients suffering from trapped lung rarely benefit from simple fluid removal, which itself often causes severe pain, dyspnea, or cough (Velardocchio et al. 1984). Since the lung is trapped, preventing reexpansion, pleurodesis is frequently impossible.
3. Fluid must reaccumulate quickly and the amount of fluid drawn off in one or several attempts must be large: like Adler and Rappole (1967), we consider a total of 2–3 liters as a minimum before considering pleurodesis.

If these three conditions above are satisfied, then pleurodesis should be seriously considered.

These criteria, in fact, do not apply only to malignant pleural exudates (Kaine 1985). Some cardiac and cirrhotic transudates (Audier et al. 1967; Davidoff et al. 1983) stubbornly persist in spite of aggressive therapy. In the latter case, the injection of radioactive tracers into ascitic fluid may show whether there is a direct leak from the peritoneal cavity to the pleural space (Verreault et al. 1986), in which case pleurodesis will have a good chance of success. However, special attention must be paid to the patient's blood pressure and intravascular volume which are often unstable due to hypoalbuminemia, as well as to the serum electrolytes, which are disturbed due to the underlying disease and agressive diuretic therapy. With this cautionary note, it should be stated that talc pleurodesis has been dramatically effective in providing symptomatic relief to 30 cirrhotic or cardiac patients in our series.

Contraindications are linked to the expansibility of the lung. Trapped lung syndrome prevents effective pleurodesis especially under two sets of circumstances.

1. In bronchogenic carcinoma or in malignancies metastatic to the bronchi, reexpansion of the lung may be limited by atelectasis due to endobronchial obstruction, sometimes with associated pneumonitis, or due to the spread of cancer to the visceral pleura (Todd et al. 1980).

2. In cases of a thick, encapsulating visceral pachypleuritis, often visible on CT scan but more easily appreciated at thoracoscopy. This pachypleuritis may be a reaction to metastatic cancer or merely be a nonspecific, chronic inflammation. In either case, pleural pressures after puncture (Light et al. 1980a; Velardocchio et al. 1984) are extremely negative, less than -20 cm H_2O. Thus, the interval between the first signs of pleurisy and the day when induced pleurodesis is considered greatly influences the chances that pleurodesis can effectively be induced, because success depends on the size of the tumor on the pleural surface and the degree of thickening of the visceral pleura.

A trapped lung is unlikely to return to a position against the chest wall, the essential requirement for pleurodesis (Fig. 55). Furthermore, attempting pleurodesis is hazardous under these circumstances for the following reasons: (a) if prolonged tube drainage is performed with the hope of slowly reexpanding the lung, the risk of secondary empyema is increased; (b) prolonged drainage further debilitates the patient by removing large amounts of proteins; and (c) the highly negative aspiration pressures risk distortion of the mediastinum on the side being drained.

Contraindications in relation to general health are a matter of clinical common sense: short life expectancy due to extreme old age or due to concomitant disease; general debilitation (Karnofski index <60). Bony metastases per se should not be an absolute contraindication, however, since local radiotherapy may provide long-term relief.

A

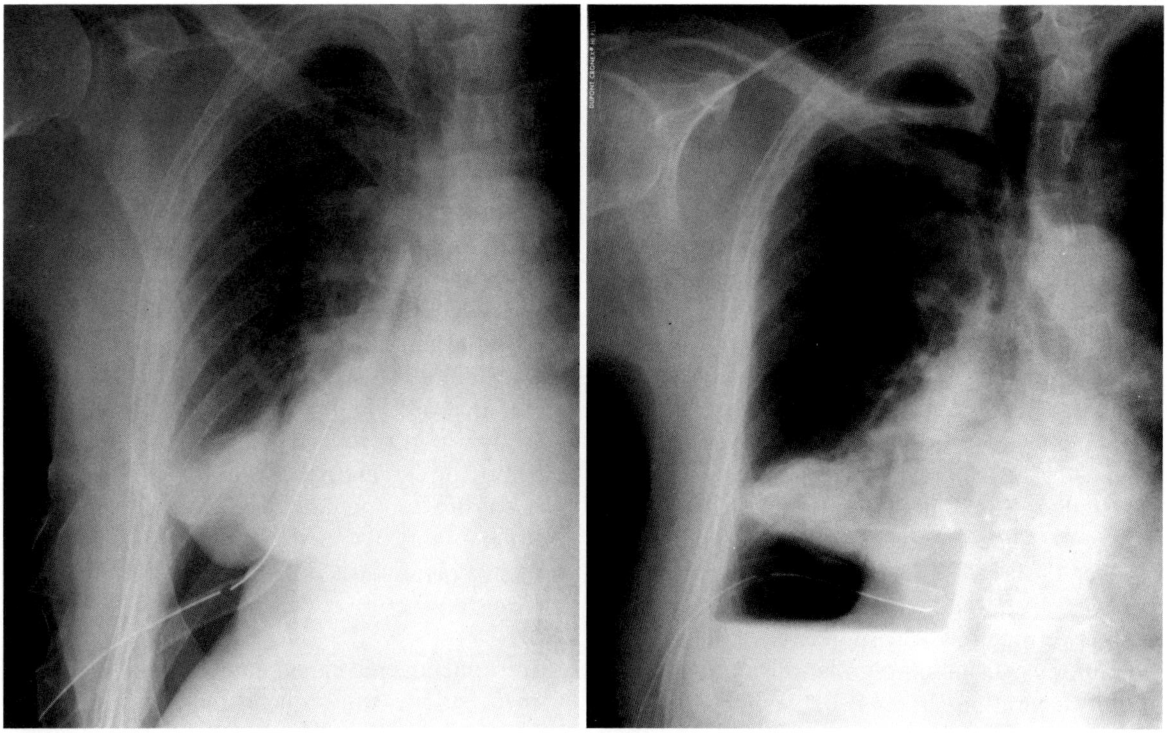

B

Fig. 55 A, B. Trapped lung: drainage difficulties. This patient presented with malignant effusion and pulmonary metastases on the right lower lobe. 1.5 liters of bloody fluid were aspirated. After puncture, the pressure was very negative (-35 cm H_2O). **A** The lung did not reexpand after two days of aspiration, **B** Even after changing the position of the drain, the lung is still a long way from the chest wall

6.2 Is Drainage of the Effusion a Necessity?

In order to obtain close contact between the parietal and visceral pleural surfaces, these patients must have a chest tube of sufficient diameter (28 to 32 Fr: Miller and Sahn 1987a, 1987b) to evacuate all exudates, including hemorrhagic exudates rich in fibrin (Good et al. 1978b).

All the substances used to induce pleurodesis are pleural irritants which produce a sclerosing effect. They destroy the layer of mesothelial cells (Thorsrud 1965), and induce pleural fibrosis (Bethune 1935; Antony 1987), which binds the visceral and parietal pleural surfaces together. This process stops the constant dripping of fluid from the pleural surface.

However, before the fibrotic bond is established, the pleural sclerosant causes a fibrinonecrotic exudate for several days (Jones 1969), which must be evacuated through the chest tube to maintain continuous contact between the pleural surfaces (Anderson et al. 1974; Fracchia et al. 1970; Rioseco 1980); then the collagenous fibrosis gradually invades the pleura. If this fibrosis is suppressed by urokinase or heparin, the action of tetracycline, for instance, is inhibited (Sahn and Good 1981).

Pleural drainage (Fig. 32) should thus be continued for several days. In a randomized study of 40 patients (Boutin et al. 1985b), we compared the use of tetracycline and talc in inducing pleurodesis. Drainage was continued until less than 100 ml was collected in a 24-h period: With talc this required 5.4 ± 3.3 days, and with tetracycline 7.0 ± 3.0 days. Total fluid evacuated was 0.8 ± 0.9 liters after talc and 1.3 ± 1.1 liters after tetracycline. Thus, talc appears to allow for a shorter hospital stay than tetracycline.

In the trapped lung syndrome, surgical decortication with or without pleurectomy, may be considered (Beattie 1963; Jensik et al. 1963; Light 1983, 1985; Weissberg and Kaufman 1980b). Sclerosants are sometimes injected intraoperatively, at the surgeon's discretion.

6.3 Deloculation of the Pleural Fluid is Often Useful

Chronic effusions are generally tapped several times, which sometimes results in the formation of multiple localized pleural fluid collections (loculations). These pockets of fluid are often difficult to tap with a needle unless multiple attempts are made, sometimes with ultrasonic or CT scan guidance. *They can be opened and drained under direct vision,* however, through the thoracoscope. Most adhesions seen are slack, fibrinous, with little vascularity, and break easily on contact with the forceps. When they are wide and thick they should be left in place, as they already ensure partial adherence of the lung to the chest wall.

While still under direct vision, the best possible position for the chest tube can be chosen; the tube must evacuate as much of the effusion as possible. If there are large adhesions partitioning the cavity, the practitioner may decide to place two tubes for drainage, usually a posteroinferior tube inserted through the seventh intercostal space and directed toward the back; and an anterior tube in the fifth or sixth intercostal space positioned high and towards the front.

As a general rule, however, one tube, of 28–32 Fr, is sufficient. It is inserted through the seventh intercostal space in the midaxillary line, reaching as high as possible (Figs. 32B, 33). After additional lateral openings are cut into it, the tube is placed either in the axillary region or even better, in the costovertebral gutter. The lowest opening, closest to the point of entry of the tube, is much more important than the others. Indeed, once aspiration has brought the lung back against the chest wall (which requires minutes to a few hours), the distal openings tend to become occluded with coagulum. The subsequent drainage will occur via the lowest opening, which therefore must be as close as feasible to the lowest point of the pleural space; above this point the effusion will be well drained, while some retained fluid often remains below it.

6.4 Sclerosing Agents

Some excellent publications have critically reviewed the gamut of methods used to induce pleurodesis (Chahinian 1985; Greenwald et al. 1978; Hausheer and Yarbro 1985; Light 1983): the interested reader may wish to peruse this material, which will not be discussed in detail here. We have chosen to emphasize only randomized studies which permit a basis for comparison (Table 4). Nonrandomized studies often suffer serious methodological problems; we will also ignore some other good studies where small numbers of patients limit their general applicability.

Among the many sclerosants which are used, only three clearly stand out: talc, tetracycline, and bleomycin. Less often used are biological products with immunological activity, such as Corynebacterium parvum (Rossi 1987). From Table 4 it is clear that simple drainage, thiotepa, and nitrogen mustard are not very effective. Tetracycline is as active as quinacrine, but the latter was poorly tolerated by patients and has been, therefore, withdrawn from general use. Bleomycin seems as active as tetracycline, but because of its reputation for inducing pulmonary fibrosis when given intravenously, it is considered potentially hazardous; Hausheer and Yarbro (1985) consider bleomycin to actually be the more active of the two. Talc is superior to tetracycline; their respective morbidity profiles are discussed in some detail below (see Tables 5, 6).

The methods of administering tetracycline and bleomycin are fairly simple. After draining the pleural space for a few days with a chest tube, the drug is injected through the tube, which is then clamped for 1-2 h; during this time the position of the patient on the bed is sequentially changed at regular intervals, with the goal of spreading the medication over the entire surface of pleura (however, a recent study using a radioactive tetracycline tracer has raised doubts as to the need for this maneuver (Lorch 1988)). The chest tube is then reconnected to the water seal, with negative pressure generally added for 48-72 h (Good and Sahn 1978a). Altogether, drainage lasts about 5-6 days, or even longer in some series: 12 days for Muir et al. (1987a, 1987b).

The effect of the sclerosant varies with the dose: the minimum dosage for tetracycline is 20 mg/kg, but this can be increased or repeated on subsequent days (Franck et al. 1989). As for bleomycin, 100 mg can be injected on the first day, followed by 200 mg on subsequent days. The patient's tolerance of this technique is generally acceptable if prior systemic analgesia is provided and topical xylocaine is injected into the chest tube at the same time as the sclerosant. Nevertheless, some patients demand large doses of narcotics after tetracycline (Harbecke 1980; Sherman 1988).

Though the duration of symphysis is an important criterion in the evaluation of the technique, it is often reported in insufficient detail for criti-

Table 4. Results of the principal randomized, controlled studies of pleurodesis in the treatment of pleurisy

	Patients (*n*)	Agents used	Success rates (%)
Mejer et al. (1977)	25	Quinacrine/Thiot[b]	64/27
Bayly et al. (1978)	22	TCN/quinacrine	83/90
Gupta et al. (1980)	25	TCN/bleomycine	58/54
Millar et al. (1980)	21	Cory/mustine	56/42
O'Neill et al. (1980)	24	TCN/drainage	72/36
Fentiman et al. (1983)	37	Mustard/talc	56/90
Zaloznik et al. (1983)	24	TCN[a]/drainage	77/22
Sorensen et al. (1984)	21	Talc/drainage	100/60
Boutin et al. (1985b)	40	Talc/TCN	90/50
Leahy et al. (1985)	32	Cory[c]/TCN	88/79
Fentiman et al. (1986)	41	Talc/TCN	92/48
Hillerdal et al. (1986)	32	Cory/bleomycine	65/13
Kessinger et al. (1987)	34	TCN/bleomycine	39/31
Muir et al. (1987b)	30	Talc/doxycycline	90/63

[a] TCN, tetracycline; [b] Thiot, thiotepa; [c] Cory, corynebacterium parvum

Table 5. Results of tetracycline pleurodesis in pleural effusions

	Patient success (*n*)	Success rate %
Rubinson and Bolooki (1972)	10/12	83
Wallach (1975)	7/7	100
Bayly et al. (1978)	10/12	83
Dunkel (1986)	53/60	80
Gravelyn et al. (1987)	15/25	60
Sherman et al. (1987)	101/108	94

The duration of successful pleural symphysis is not always described. Since tetracycline is soluble, it may be reabsorbed and its action might have a limited duration

Table 6. Results of talc pleurodesis in pleural effusions

		Patient success (*n*)	Success rate (%)
Prorok and Nealon (1968)	Thoracotomy	39/43	90
Haupt et al. (1960)	Thoracotomy	19/19	100
Chambers (1958)	Thoracotomy or Thoracentesis	19/20	85
Pizzocaro et al. (1973)	Thoracotomy or Thoracoscopy	18/23	78
Pearson and Mac Gregor (1966)	Thoracentesis or Thoracotomy	13/17	76
Jones (1969)	Thoracoscopy	20/21	95
Adler and Rappole (1967)	Thoracentesis	4/4	100
Roche et al. (1963)	Thoracoscopy	6/6	100
Todd et al. (1980)	Thoracotomy or Thoracentesis	158/163	90
Scarbonchi et al. (1981)	Thoracoscopy	67/77	87
Weissberg et al. (1980a)	Thoracoscopy	34/39	87
Harley (1979)	Thoracoscopy	40/44	90
Shedbalkar et al. (1971)	Thoracoscopy	22/28	79
Aherne (1982)	Thoracoscopy	18/25	72
Escamilla et al. (1986)	Thoracoscopy	80/99	80
Canto et al. (1985a)	Thoracoscopy	110/128	86
Boniface and Guerin (1989)	Thoracoscopy	251/270	93
Ladjimi et al. (1989)	Thoracoscopy	170/218	78

cal review. Sometimes a "complete response" is described when, in fact, the duration of the response was limited. A fair definition of "complete response" should require that follow-up for a stated period of time confirmed the *persistence* of the pleural symphysis. In our study (Boutin et al. 1985b), tetracycline gave good initial results in 90% of the patients, but 50% relapsed within 6 months (Fig. 56). This pattern was also the case for:

1. Ostrowski (1986): 69% responses at 1 month but only 54% at 3 months
2. Gravelyn et al. (1987): 16% had lasting success, 44% had a moderate recurrence of fluid, and 40% had sufficient recurrence to require further drainage
3. Dunkel (1986): 28 out of 60 patients had a late recurrence
4. Sherman et al. (1987): 94% with initial response, but 49% had recurrence of symptoms at 3 months.

As tetracycline and bleomycin are soluble, it is possible that they gradually disappear from the pleural cavity: Wooten et al. (1987) noted that 96 min after a pleural injection of 20 mg/kg, the blood levels of tetracycline were 3.6 ± 0.9 µg/ml. In contrast, talc is insoluble and will remain in place indefinitely, bringing about permanent pleurodesis (Shedbalkar et al. 1971).

Talc poudrage (Fig. 57) seems to us one of the best methods: in our series of 300 patients, we achieved satisfactory, permanent pleurodesis in 90% of all cases of malignant pleurisy. We also matched 14 mesothelioma patients who underwent thoracoscopic talc poudrage with 14 others undergoing thoracotomy and pleurectomy: there was no difference in terms of effusion suppres-

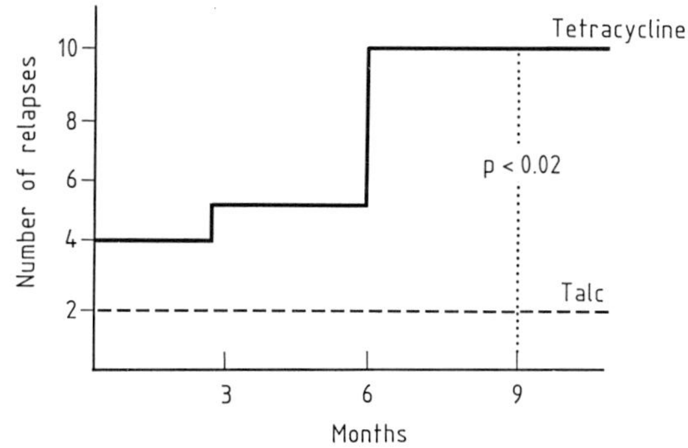

Fig. 56. Relapses after talc versus tetracycline pleurodesis. 40 patients with malignant pleural effusion were randomly chosen for either talc or tetracycline instillation under thoracoscopy (Boutin et al. 1985b). There is no significant difference between talc and tetracycline during the first month. As the months pass, however, talc pleurodesis persists whereas relapses occur in patients treated with tetracycline

sion or survival (Scarbonchi et al. 1981). This result, which has been reproduced in Frankel's animal model (Frankel et al. 1961), has been confirmed by most randomized studies (see Table 4), and several general reviews (Fentiman 1987; Greenwald et al. 1978; Hausheer and Yarbro 1985). We share the opinion of Hausheer and Yarbro, for whom "it seems likely that talc represents the most effective sclerosing agent available, even after other agents have failed to control effusion."

On the other hand, some reports have decried talc pleurodesis, suggesting unacceptable morbidity (Gaensler 1956; Hausheer and Yarbro 1985). Deaths have been reported soon after talc poudrage (Pearson and MacGregor 1966), but this seems to be due to factors of patient selection: these cases were already in the late stages of cancer, and had a very limited life expectancy in any case. Three cases of acute respiratory failure after 10 g of talc saline suspension were instilled were reported by Rinaldo et al. (1983). Todd et al. (1980) observed seven cases of respiratory failure and/or pneumonia, in a series of 146 patients, but no precise details are provided. We believe these reports overstate the risk. Only once did we observe pulmonary edema in 300 consecutive talc poudrages, and this one case was clearly related to overly rapid pleural fluid aspiration in a patient with far-advanced cancer (Boutin et al. 1986a).

With patients selected according to the criteria described above, we experienced no other serious problems, and talc tolerance was the same as in patients receiving tetracycline. There is, however, an important difference in pain perception when dealing with spontaneous pneumothorax, where the pleural surfaces are perfectly healthy and react violently in response to any foreign body contact. Chronic effusions produce pleural thickening which is associated with decreased pain response, so that talc poudrage, applied un-

A

B

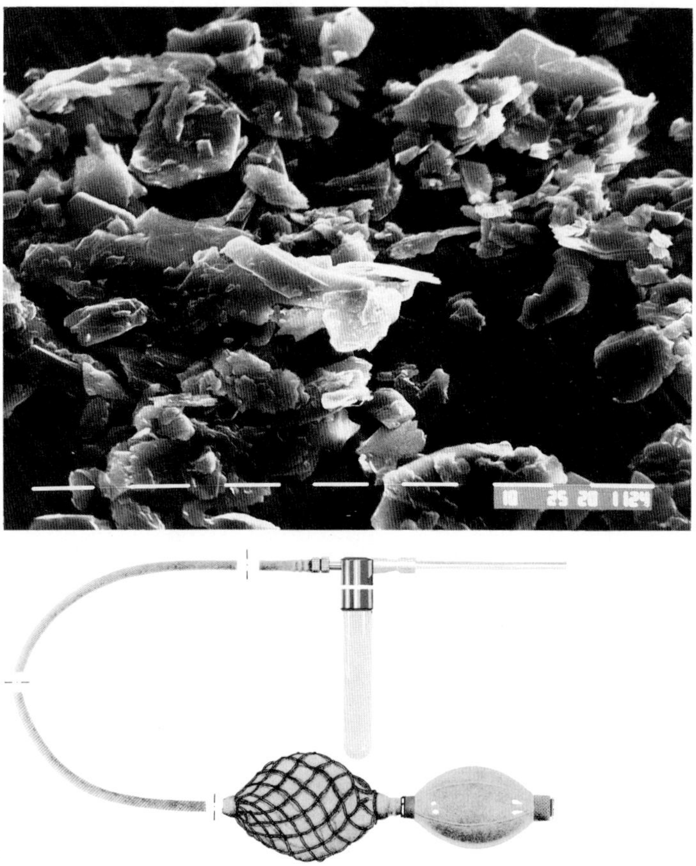

Fig. 57 A, B. Talc. **A** Luzenac talc (France) contains no fibers. Electon microscope photograph (× 1024). **B** A talc atomizer

der local anesthesia, is relatively painless. This is in sharp contrast to the severe pain after tetracycline instillation, a pain that intra-pleural xylocaine and high doses of parenteral narcotics do not always relieve.

In long-term follow-up, we have never encountered the extensive pleural fibrosis described by Gaensler (1956), nor any chronic residual pain or other late complications. This is probably the result of our judicious use of talc (no more than 6-9 ml - 3-4.5 g - are instilled), and to our strict attention to complete fluid drainage in the days following talcage.

Tetracycline is currently considered to be the sclerosant of choice (Antony et al. 1985a, 1985b, 1987; Chahinian 1985) whereas talc is deemed "old fashioned". True enough, talc poudrage requires more equipment than tetracycline instillation, and some familiarity with thoracoscopy (talc instillation has been much less effective when attempted without thoracoscopy, in saline suspension, for example). Nevertheless, we feel talc is the sclerosant of first choice because of its greater effectiveness and greater permanency, even without considering the pain endured by the patient with tetracycline (Boutin 1989c). When tetracycline is used first, but fails, the indication for talc is even greater (Austin and Flye 1979; Hausheer and Yarbro 1985; Leff et al. 1978; Muir et al. 1987a). The alternative of trying tetracycline a second time should probably be discouraged.

6.5 Newer Agents for Pleurodesis, Including Bioadhesives

Corynebacterium parvum has been used for pleurodesis by several authors (Mc Leod et al. 1985; Webb et al. 1978); its efficacy is similar to that of tetracycline (Leahy et al. 1985) and nitrogen mustard (Millar et al. 1980), and is reported to be superior to that of bleomycin by Hillerdal et al. (1986). New and interesting immunological effects were expected; in fact, its only action seems to be related to a simple increase in polymorphonucleocytes (Rossi et al. 1987), which generate fibrosis as do any other agents used for pleural symphysis.

Beta-interferon instilled intraperitoneally was studied by Rambaldi et al. (1985) in ovarian cancer cases; Weimar et al. (1981) used it in pleural mesotheliomas. Besides its antitumor activity, interferon also stimulates proliferation of fibroblasts, according to Hunninghake at al. (1986). In a series of 25 pleural mesotheliomas, we tested intrapleural gamma interferon, instilling 40 million units 16 times over a 2-month period: we observed a complete response histopathologically proven in six out of ten patients with stage I mesothelioma (to be published).

After some preliminary results had been reported (Ottow et al. 1987) studies based on the intrapleural instillation of interleukin 2 are in progress in our department.

Kreuser et al. (1985) have tested fibrin glue in 27 patients. They injected 2000 units of aprotinin, 10 ml of fibrinogen, and 10 ml of thrombin in the pleural space. Complete pleurodesis was achieved in 19 of these, and 2 more had partial success. Preliminary studies in dogs in our department, however, failed to achieve pleural symphysis (Seitz et al. 1989).

6.6 Conclusion

In the many patients with indication for pleurodesis, there are three reasons for using thoracoscopy (Oakes et al. 1984):

1. To remove partitions from the pleural cavity, eliminating pockets of fluid which are inaccessible to simple puncture (and thereby to sclerosants), and which have considerable radiological and functional consequences (McLoud 1980). This reduces a multilocular space to a unilocular one, much easier to drain. This may also allow the lung to return to its most functional position.
2. Under direct vision, one can choose the best point of entry for the chest tube and the best location to leave the tube, guaranteeing optimal drainage.
3. To pulverize 3-4.5 g of talc under direct vision,

insuring that all surfaces are covered. Performed in this way, talc poudrage has the best record in achieving complete and persistent pleurodesis. Suspension of talc in saline is not comparable and may be hazardous.

Chapter 7: Thoracoscopy in the Diagnosis and Treatment of Spontaneous Pneumothorax

7.1 Indications for Thoracoscopy

Since no one course of action has been established as the state of the art for spontaneous pneumothorax, discussion often evokes passionate arguments among pulmonologists. This results partly from the varied estimations of risk for spontaneous recurrences, which vary from 20%–50%, and the fact that a certain amount of personal judgment is often involved in selecting therapy. The statement that 28% of pneumothoraces relapse after a first episode (Table 10) can be interpreted in two ways: the conservative physician could claim a permanent cure in 72% of the cases; the more interventionist surgeon would say that a 28% risk of relapse, sometimes under hazardous conditions, is not acceptable since safe methods of inducing pleurodesis are available.

The truth is that the actual percentage of relapse is not exactly known. In an epidemiological study, Melton et al. (1979) estimated the occurrence of a first episode to be 8.6/100000 and that of a second episode to be 8.3/100000, with no significant difference between the two figures; the number of relapses, therefore, appears to be high.

Relapses are unpredictable; they are, of course, linked to the presence of bullae and blebs on the surface of the lung. The size of these lesions has been classified by L. Reid (1967) as follows:

Type 1: small bullae and blebs which are only visible under the light microscope
Type 2: more voluminous bullae which are sessile and communicate with adjacent lung parenchyma
Type 3: very large bullae.

Under electronic microscopy one can see pores on the visceral pleura measuring 10–20 μm in diameter in the places where mesothelial cells were previously seen (elastofibrosis), and which are responsible for the air leak (Ohata and Suzuli 1980). These pores cannot be seen by the naked eye, explaining perhaps why Sattler (1937) stated that there were cases of pneumothorax where the visceral pleura appeared to be intact. Nonetheless, in most cases there are macroscopic lesions on the surface of the lung. When they are small, however, they cannot be recognized on roentgenograms or CT scan. The study of such lesions is, therefore, one of the applications of thoracoscopy.

The surgeon is called upon to resect some emphysematous bullae and to cauterize blebs; if the lesions are localized, the thoracoscopist can also do this using a Nd:YAG laser or electrocautery, thus avoiding a thoracotomy. The goal of preventing recurrent pneumothorax may generally be achieved without thoracotomy, by medical pleurodesis performed via thoracoscopy. As Thomas and Gebauer (1958) remarked, emphysematous bullae and blebs are often congenital and due in part to hypovascularization of the peripheral pulmonary parenchyma; pleurodesis encourages new vessels to form and might stop these lesions from developing.

Finally, lesions evolve with age (Ohata and Suzuli 1980; Reid 1967), and it is better to diagnose and treat them in their early stages than to wait until they are more developed.

In our department, the placement of a chest tube is always accompanied by a quick thoracoscopic examination, rapidly performed with 4-mm Panoview direct and oblique telescopes introduced by the same orifice as the chest tube. Three obvious benefits are provided: (a) the lesions are precisely assessed under direct vision;

(b) the best location for the chest tube may be found; and (c) for teaching purposes, the thoracic organs can be seen best in a spontaneous pneumothorax, where the pleura is thin and transparent. This is a practical opportunity for the young pulmonologist to learn his or her way around the thoracic cavity and to gain confidence in handling the various instruments.

To summarize, indications for thoracoscopy in pneumothorax are the same as for chest tube insertion for drainage. That is to say:

1. To reduce the pneumothorax, especially when large, recurrent, chronic; when associated with fluid, blood, pus or with high pressure.
2. Whenever pleurodesis is indicated: in respiratory insufficiency, with silicosis, in recurrent catamenial pneumothorax, in histiocytosis X, with pulmonary fibrosis, etc. In these cases, medical pleurodesis is less invasive and provides less pain, discomfort or sequelae than thoracotomy.

7.2 Thoracoscopic Findings in Spontaneous Pneumothorax

Sattler was the first, in 1937, to identify emphysematous bullae under thoracoscopic view in spontaneous pneumothorax. In his series, ruptured bullae were identified in 63% of the patients, whereas no evident bullae or air leaks were seen in the others. Bullous perforations were subsequently reported by others (Benda and Aubin 1955). Thoracoscopic studies in Utrecht, the Netherlands, by Swierenga et al. (1974, 1977) and Wagenaar (1970) were confirmed by Vanderschueren (1981a). Among 126 patients, he distinguished the following four stages of spontaneous pneumothorax:

Stage I: idiopathic pneumothorax, the lung being endoscopically normal: 40% of cases
Stage II: pneumothorax with pleuro-pulmonary adhesions: 12%
Stage III: pneumothorax with small bullae and blebs, less than 2 cm in diameter: 31%
Stage IV: pneumothorax with numerous large bullae more than 2 cm in diameter: 17% (Table 7).

Stage I pneumothorax. The lung appears normal when the usual telescopes are used. The fissures, which are opened for inspection, and the mediastinal side of the lung seem also normal.

However, modern magnifying telescopes (Panoview) and video recordings make it possible to see details which could not be appreciated using older telescopes: minute blebs and small emphysematous bullae, about 1–2 mm in diameter, are seen to be the cause of the pneumothorax. Thus it can be said that there is no such thing as a thoracoscopically normal lung in patients with a "idiopathic" spontaneous pneumothorax. These lesions are too fine to be seen on CT scan (Figs. 19, 58). They are certainly too small for surgical resection. However, our ability to detect lesions endoscopically mandates that action be taken to correct the defects and prevent further recurrences. The conservative approach of chest tube insertion, water-seal drainage, and rest seems to us inadequate, considering the known high frequency of recurrence.

We usually induce pleurodesis in these patients by thoracoscopic dusting of no more than 2–3 ml of talc over the involved area (Table 8, Fig. 59). Other authors describe the use of biological adhesives or tetracycline for this purpose.

Stage II pneumothorax. Adhesions are commonplace in the pleural cavity but are seen less often

Table 7. Spontaneous Pneumothorax: distribution of endoscopic lesions according to Vanderschueren's classification

	Vanderschueren (*n*=126) (%)	Guerin (*n*=109) (%)	Our series (*n*=100) (%)
Type I[a]	40	30	30
Type II	12	13	12
Type III	31	28	41
Type IV	17	29	17

If high magnification (×4 to ×9) photographs and video recordings connected to a lens with a long focal length are used during thoracoscopy, pulmonary lesions can be seen which are too small to be recognized using an ordinary lens: one can almost always find bubbles and/or blebs at stage I. Realistically, it might be asked whether the lung is ever normal in cases of spontaneous pneumothorax.

[a] Using normal telescope and lens

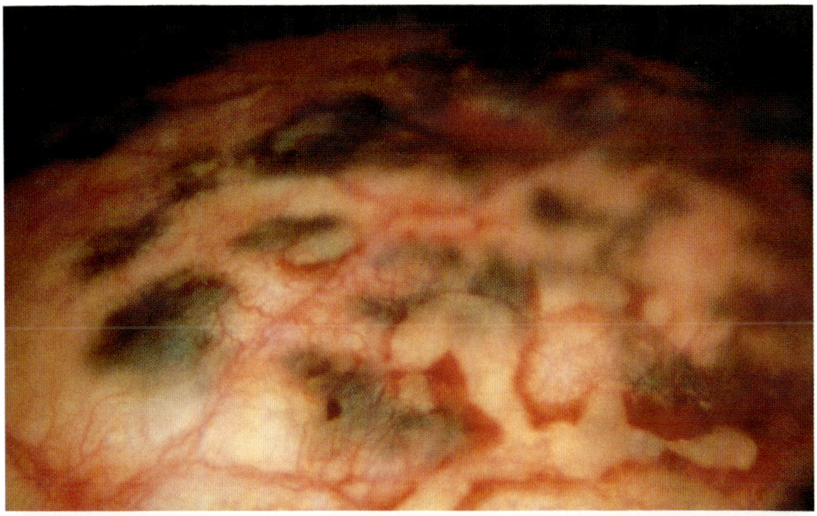

Fig. 58. Small blebs in spontaneous pneumothorax. The blebs on this photo are less than 2 mm in diameter, and can only be seen under thoracoscopy with a high-quality optical magnification. One can see pulmonary anthracotic pigment delimiting the pulmonary lobules, as well as the fine ramifications of the pulmonary veins on the surface

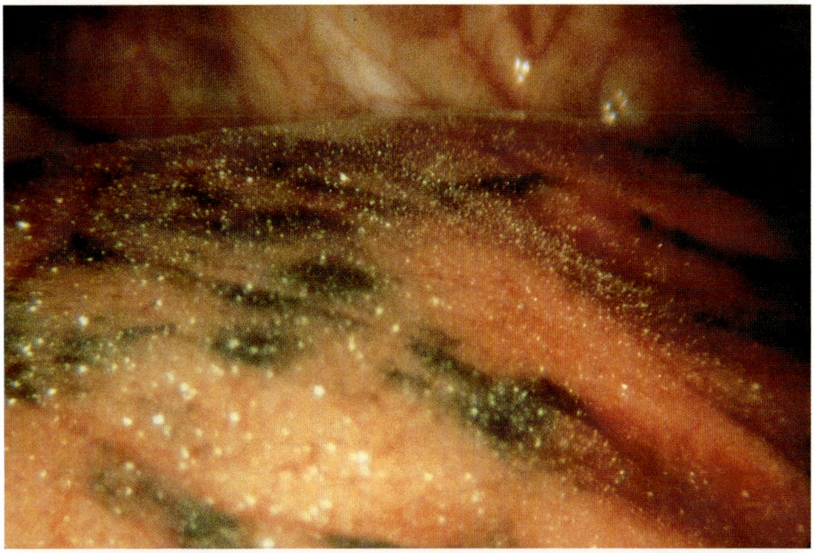

Fig. 59. Talc poudrage in spontaneous pneumothorax. This patient suffered from recurrent pneumothorax. There was no further recurrence after talc poudrage and 3 days of pleural drainage

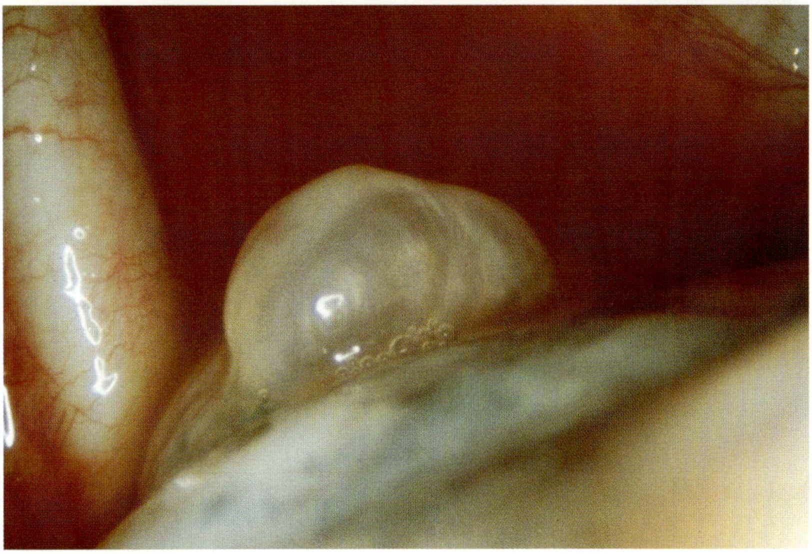

Fig. 60. Spontaneous pneumothorax: blebs. Typical, 1 cm bleb: the visceral pleura is detached from the lung, creating this blister with a very thin, nonvascularized wall; it is translucent and very fragile. These lesions appear frequently on the apical surface of the lung. The subclavian artery can be seen on the *left* in the background

in spontaneous pneumothorax than in cases of pleural effusion: this lack of adhesions partially explains the great number of recurrences.

Moreover, adhesions may result from chest tube drainage during a previous episode of pneumothorax. The adhesions are situated along the tube tract, separating the pleural cavity into two separate chambers but not preventing a subsequent air leak.

Adhesions can make exploration of the pleural cavity difficult; if necessary, some of them can be divided. In some cases, a ruptured emphysematous bulla is situated at the foot of the adhesion, which holds it open; severing this adhesion permits the pleural defect to close. At the same time the defect may be sealed with a biological adhesive, or it can be coagulated using a laser which shrinks the visceral pleura, thus closing the defect. A spontaneously torn adhesion can be the

Table 8. Thoracoscopy in spontaneous pneumothorax stage-related algorithm

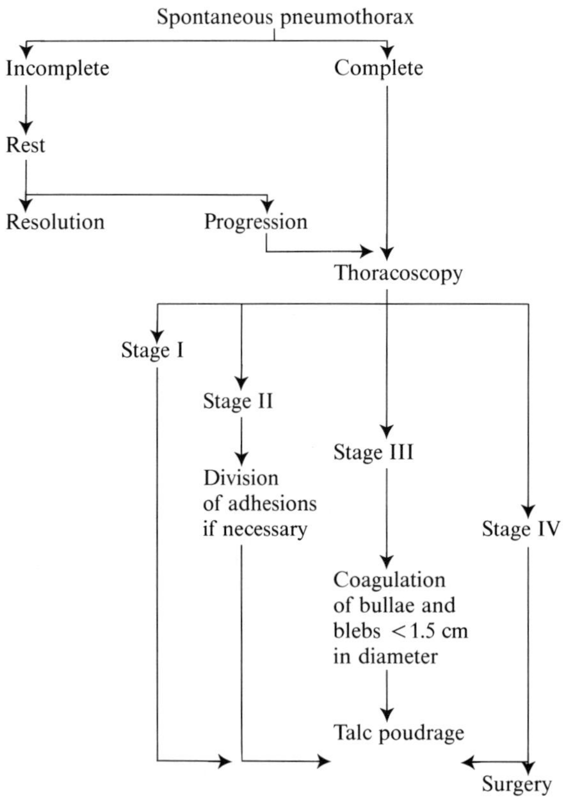

A pleural drain is always inserted under direct vision. Pulmonary lesions are found in almost every patient but often require optical magnification to be seen

cause of an hemorrhage complicating a pneumothorax; coagulating the bleeding vessel will stem the hemorrhage.

With these few exceptions, there is no point in attacking these adhesions.

Stage III pneumothorax. Obvious emphysematous lesions can be seen on the surface of the lung. Blebs (Fig. 60) have a very thin avascular wall, are transparent, and vary in size from less than 1 mm on up, but rarely exceed 1 cm in diameter. There are no direct communications with the alveoli and bronchioles. They can be coagulated only if not more than 1.5–2.0 cm in diameter, or if they are thin and pedunculated at their base (Kaiser 1989c).

These smaller lesions, therefore, are accessible to thoracoscopic treatment: coagulation, followed by medical pleurodesis. The end results are similar to those of surgical pleurodesis, but the patient is spared of having to undergo a thoracotomy.

Stage IV pneumothorax. This stage is characterized by dystrophic bullous changes, with numerous bullae and blebs over 2 cm in diameter (Figs. 61, 62). Optimal treatment for these lesions is surgical resection. Therefore, we often merely place a drainage tube and transfer the patient to the surgical wards. On the other hand, we may perform talc poudrage in cases where surgery is contraindicated, for instance in respiratory failure due to severe chronic bronchitis or any other far-advanced pulmonary disease. Sometimes a ruptured pedunculated bulla can be coagulated without any difficulty (Fig. 63).

During thoracoscopy, the visibility of bullae and blebs can be enhanced if the patient can perform a Valsalva maneuver, or by creating positive airway pressure with the anesthesia mask. The previously flattened, invisible bubbles then project from the surface of the lung. Conversely, positive pressure from the pleural side may also bring out the bubbles: air is gradually instilled through the thoracoscope, forcing the lung to collapse; the collapse is greatest in the healthy areas, while air imprisoned in the bullae and blebs makes them stand out on the surface. A way to find any air leakage is to make the patient breathe an aerosol of Fluorescéine for about

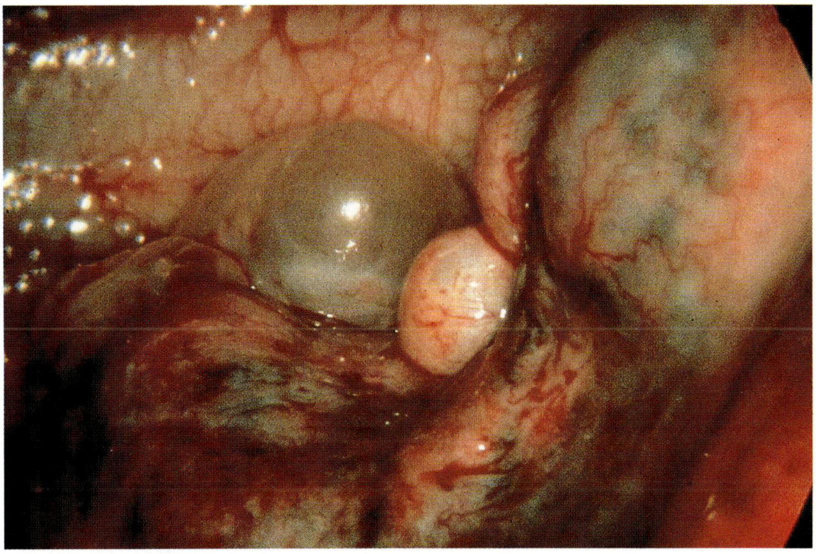

Fig. 61. Spontaneous pneumothorax: bullous dystrophy of the apex. The surface of the pulmonary apex is completely covered with emphysematous bullae and blebs which are easy to differentiate; they vary in size from 0.5 to 2 cm in diameter. At the *bottom*, part of the lung is normal. In the background, the parietal pleura

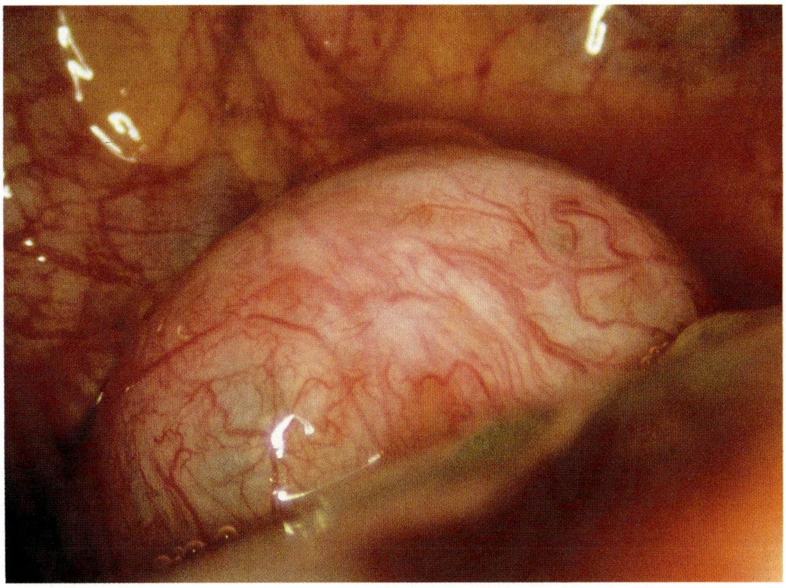

Fig. 62. Spontaneous pneumothorax: emphysematous bulla. This emphysematous bulla looks very different from a bleb; it has a thick, opaque, highly vascularized surface, rather like pulmonary parenchyma. This bulla is 2.5 cm in diameter. In this case, it is an isolated finding on the lung, is sessile, and has not been coagulated; the patient received talc poudrage

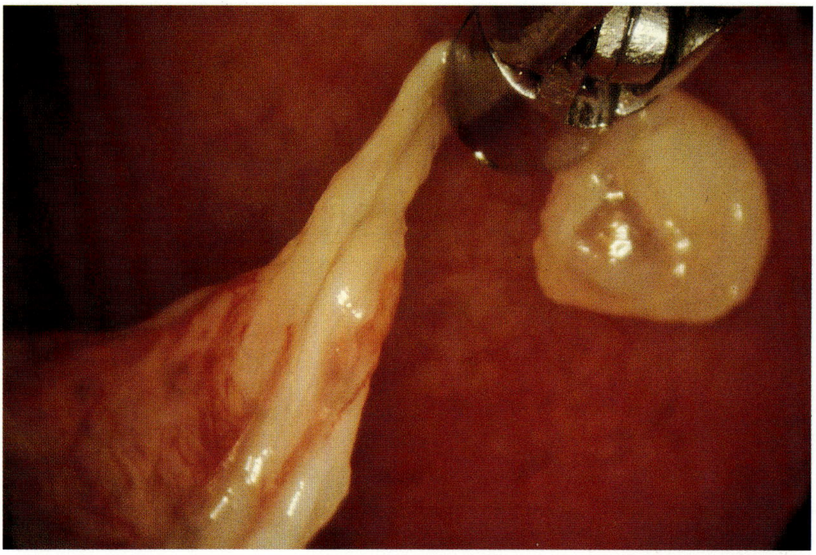

Fig. 63. Spontaneous pneumothorax: rupture of a large emphysematous bulla. This patient, aged 62, had chronic respiratory insufficiency, with bilateral emphysematous bullae seen on X-ray. A spontaneous pneumothorax induced respiratory failure, with hypoxemia that decreased from 62 to 50 Torr. Thoracoscopy showed a large, ruptured bulla (here lifted with the forceps) that was easily coagulated

20 min prior to thoracoscopy; the leak will appear yellowish during thoracoscopic examination.

The size of bullous lesions correlates with age: A review of 87 patients showed a good correlation between the patient's age and the size of the lesions (Table 9). Most patients in stage IV were over 40 years old and suffered from chronic bronchitis, some of them having respiratory insufficiency. Thus, several patients received talc poudrage instead of undergoing surgery.

Table 9. Spontaneous pneumothorax: age distribution of patients according to Vanderschueren's stages

Stage[a]	Number	Average age (years)
I	24	25
III	47	32
IV	16	46.5
	87	

The age of patients in stage IV is significantly greater than in the other stages ($p < 0.01$). Thus, there are more cases of stage I in young people, and many more cases of stage IV in those over 40.
[a] Vanderschueren (1981)

7.3 Results of Induced Pleurodesis in Spontaneous Pneumothorax

We reviewed in Table 10 the results of the different treatments proposed for spontaneous pneumothorax in 75 published series. Simple bedrest was associated with a 28% rate of recurrence. Chest tube drainage with 21% recurrences and thoracotomy with only 1.5% recurrences, but this low rate is not achieved without morbidity and complications.

Results of the various methods of medical pleurodesis are as follows:

1. *Tetracycline:* 10 published series included 202 patients, of whom 20% relapsed. Larger studies with long-term follow-up need to be performed before any definitive conclusions may be drawn. A randomized study conducted by Light (personal communication, 1989) compared two groups of patients, one receiving tetracycline, and the other simple drainage: his results clearly showed the benefit of tetracycline, albeit with over 20% eventual recurrences.

   Since tetracycline is soluble, an important

question is whether the pleural symphysis endures for years after the drug has withdrawn from the thorax. Tetracycline, like talc, can be quite painful in patients without pleural thickening.

2. *Fibrin glue* has been used in 8 series: 15% relapses were recorded. A study in our department (Seitz et al. 1989) showed that Tissucol did not cause pleural fibrosis in dogs: the mesothelium was indeed intact, and the pleura peeled away easily at autopsy. Nevertheless, the idea of a biological glue devoid of side effects remains intriguing; hopefully, further refinements in the methodology of this approach will lead to greater efficacy.
3. *Talc:* in 505 patients from 13 published series the number of relapses was only 7%, with even lower percentages in the three largest studies (Guerin et al. 1985b; Vanderschueren 1981a; Boutin et al. 1985). In the most recent study, Viskum et al. (1989b) reexamined 99 patients 22 to 35 years after talc poudrage for idiopathic spontaneous pneumothorax; only 2.5% had had a relapse.

The number of relapses is thus similar to that observed after thoracotomy. The effectiveness of talc is actually not in question, either in humans or in animal models (Bethune 1935; Frankel et al. 1961; Seitz et al. 1989). However, talc, like tetracycline, is not easy to tolerate in patients who generally have no chronic pleural thickening. Effective analgesics must be given prior to dusting the talc in order to minimize the immediate discomfort caused by contact with the powder and by the reexpansion of the lung to the chest wall during tube drainage. Fortunately, this discomfort generally lasts only a few minutes, which is much shorter than the period of pain from tetracycline injected into the cavity.

Post-thoracoscopic drainage. In our department, chest tube drainage lasted an average of 5.6 days, with the majority of patients being extubated after only 3-4 days.

Concerns about talc. Using talc in young patients with a benign disease such as spontaneous pneu-

Table 10. Spontaneous pneumothorax relapse rates after various treatments (compiled from 75 published series)

Treatment	Series *(n)*	Source[a]	Years	Total cases *(n)*	Failure/relapse (average %)
Rest	13	1	1961-1983	912	28
Drainage	13	2	1961-1989	1627	21
Cyclines	10	3	1982-1989	202	20
Fibrin glue	8	4	1978-1987	493	15.2
Talc	13	5	1947-1989	505	7.3
Talc (personal series)			1985	100	5
Thoracotomy	18	6	1949-1984	1143	1.5

[a] References:
1 Bernhard et al. (1962), Bonnefoy et al. (1978), Brocard et al. (1961), Givel et al. (1984), Hyde (1963), Lallemand and Humbert (1963), Lynn (1965), Maurel et al. (1971), Myers (1954), Smith and Rothwel (1962), Stanek et al. (1961), Stradling and Poole (1966), Wagenaar (1970).
2 Almind (1989), Bariffi et al. (1979), Bonnefoy et al. (1978), Getz and Beasley (1983), Givel et al. (1984), Lallemand and Humbert (1963), Lynn (1965), Maurel et al. (1971), Ruckley and Cormack (1966), Smith and Rothwel (1962), Stanek et al. (1961), Wagenaar (1970), Wied et al. (1981).
3 Almany and Sherman (1987), Almind (1989), Grosser et al. (1989), Krasnik et al. (1987), Morel (1984), Mortenson (1987), Olivier (1982), Senigaglia et al. (1987), Tassi (1983), Wied et al. (1983).
4 Bense (1987), Buchwald (1984), Elert and Eigel (1986), Guerin et al. (1987), Heindl and Pridun (1986), Kaiser and Wolfart (1983), Spiegel et al. (1983), Takeno (1978).
5 Almind (1989), Driscoll and Aronstam (1961), Guerin et al. (1985b), Marrangoni et al. (1955), Nandi (1980), Nico (1950), Roche (1965), Smith and Rothwel (1962), Steele (1947), Tribble et al. (1986), Vanderschueren (1981a), Viskum et al. (1989b), Weissberg et al. (1980a).
6 Driscoll and Aronstam (1961), Eschapasse et al. (1977), Gaensler (1956), Gamondes et al. (1984), Getz and Beasley (1983), Givel et al. (1984), Gobbel et al. (1963), Guibert et al. (1984), Lallemand (1963), Martigne et al. (1980), Maurel et al. (1971), Meade and Blades (1949), Ruckley and Cormack (1966), Smith and Rothwel (1962), Stanek et al. (1961), Thomas and Gebauer (1958), Viard et al. (1984), Youmans et al. (1970)

mothorax has given rise to questions about long-term safety:

Is talc poudrage carcinogenic? This concern is related to the fact that certain talcs, including the one from New Jersey, contain tremolite or asbestos, which are known carcinogens. There is no evidence linking asbestos-free pure talc, such as that used by Guerin, Vanderschueren, and us, with any malignant processes. A retrospective study published by the Research Committee of the British Thoracic Association (1979) showed that none of the subjects treated with talc over a period of 18 years showed any signs of mesothelioma. It has been suggested that a longer time span of 20–30 years should be studied. The Copenhagen study cited above (Lange 1988; Viskum et al., 1989b) found no cases of mesothelioma after a 22- to 35-year follow-up in 80 patients. In actual fact, the first treatments using talc for pneumothorax were begun by Bethune in 1933 – 57 years ago – and not a single case of mesothelioma has been published in these or any subsequent patients. On the other hand, when asbestos is dusted into the pericardium as formerly proposed to revascularize the myocardium after an infarct, malignant tumors may develop. Churg et al. (1978) reported a case of mesothelioma developing within 15 years after pericardial poudrage with asbestos. The International Agency for Research against Cancer in Lyon, in an exhaustive monograph, recently concluded that talc was not carcinogenic (I.A.R.C. 1987). Leophonte et al. (1983) reached the same conclusion in their study of a cohort of talc miners. It should be added that the international scientific community is so keen to discover any nonasbestos related causes of mesothelioma that any possible link between talc and this tumor would have been published immediately.

Is talc fibrogenic? Here, there appears to be confusion with the fibrotic action of the "talc" lubricant dusted years ago on surgeon's gloves; this "surgical powder" was actually starch mixed with calcium carbonate and contained no talc at all. The starch is implicated in progressive peritoneal granulomata which has nothing to do with the true talc under discussion here. Gaensler (1956) rejected talc because he felt it could induce fibrosis, but he gave no details and cited no reference. In fact, in all the series published on thoracoscopic use of talc, there is not one case reported of progressive pleural fibrosis. However, we cannot rule out a dose-effect relationship that might render talc fibrogenic when used at high doses (for instance if large concentrations of talc are suspended in saline and injected into the pleura).The small amounts used by us (2–3 ml) do not lead to any discernable fibrosis.

In our series, talc did not induce any permanent radiological changes in 90% of the patients in whom, indeed, it was eventually impossible to discern which side had received the poudrage. A permanent border on the pleura, some 1–3 mm thick, was developed in 5% of cases primarily at the apex. The remaining 5% had some blunting of the costophrenic angle. The roentgenographic sequelae from thoracotomy are generally much more dramatic.

The functional sequelae of talc are minor: Vanderschueren (1981a) reported almost no spirometric abnormalities. In 54 patients, Lange (1988) found a drop in total lung capacity of 7%, compared to 21 patients treated with simple tube drainage; considering that the 21 patients not given talc were most likely the milder cases, this minor difference observed probably exaggerates the real effect of talc. In a recent study, we measured alveolar clearance with ^{99}Tc D.T.P.A. before and after talc poudrage; clearance was abnormally high before thoracoscopy because of the pneumothorax but returned quickly to normal after thoracoscopy, within fourteen days. This lack of a measurable increase in the permeability of the alveolar membrane induced by talc poudrage correlates with the negative electron microscope search for talc on bronchoalveolar lavage fluid, which we carried out in three patients 1 week after talc poudrage (Boutin et al. 1988b).

7.4 Conclusion

Thoracotomy effectively prevents recurrence of spontaneous pneumothorax but is highly invasive, requires general anesthesia, causes several days or weeks of pain from the incision, leaves a large permanent scar, and cannot be performed by nonsurgically trained pulmonologists. Therefore surgery should be reserved for those patients with blebs and bullae which are too large for less invasive procedures.

Talc poudrage seems to be the more effective medical procedure in inducing pleurodesis; it has some pain associated with it, but has the highest rate of long-term success, with negligible radiographic and functional sequelae. Combining talc poudrage with thoracoscopy provides rapid identification of the cause of the leak and usually a permanent cure.

Tetracycline causes at least as much pain as talc and is probably less effective; randomized studies would be useful to discriminate advantages and shortcomings of both methods. As for fibrin glue, it shows promise and is not painful, but requires further study and improvement.

Chapter 8: Other Indications for Thoracoscopy

There are a number of relatively interesting but unfrequent indications for thoracoscopy. The thoracoscopist in training need not be concerned about these indications, as they usually require a good deal of experience. They should be mentioned, however, for the sake of completeness and to indicate the possible scope of the technique for the physician who truly becomes an expert.

8.1 Pulmonary Biopsy

There are several methods of performing pulmonary biopsies: surgical biopsy at thoracotomy (Wall et al. 1981) has become the "gold standard" of comparison, as its diagnostic results are the most sensitive and the most specific of all techniques. It is also the most invasive, however, relegating its use to occasions where simpler methods have failed.

The simplest method of "sampling the lung" is broncho-alveolar lavage (BAL), which is generally free of morbidity and risk to the patient; it is useful both diagnostically (e. g., in pneumocystis and histiocytosis X) and in understanding the basic pathophysiology of certain diseases (e. g., sarcoidosis, pulmonary fibrosis), but few histopathological diagnoses can actually be made.

Between these two extremes in the degree of invasiveness, there is wide current use of transbronchial lung biopsy through the flexible fiberoptic bronchoscope. Most large diagnostic centers are adept in percutaneous needle biopsy of the lung, using fluoroscopic control or a CT scan. Thoracoscopic biopsy provides another option (Hatch and Blalock 1966; Heine 1957).

In our department, we studied thoracoscopic lung biopsy first in animals and then in man (Boutin et al. 1982a), demonstrating a high diagnostic yield with low morbidity (Figs. 30, 64, 70).

8.1.1 Indications

There are at least five:

1. For biopsy of the visceral pleura and of the lung surface in patients with chronic pleural effusions due to mesothelioma, metastatic tumor, asbestosis, or with quickly growing asbestotic pleural plaques where associated cancer must be ruled out. The pulmonary biopsy is carried out both for diagnosis and for staging known pleural malignancies (e. g., is the mesothelioma stage IA or IB?).
2. To perform a mineralologic study of asbestos-fiber burden of the lung.
3. For single or multiple peripheral pulmonary opacities, where a transbronchial or percutaneous lung biopsy is nondiagnostic.
4. For diffuse pulmonary diseases which reach the periphery : these may be biopsied when other simpler techniques have failed to provide a diagnosis. Examples include granulomatous processes, especially sarcoidosis and invasive fungal disease, histiocytosis X, diffuse interstitial fibrosis (cryptogenic fibrosing alveolitis), silicosis, asbestosis, other pneumoconioses, collagen-vascular diseases, lymphangitic cancer, etc. (Bayle et al. 1982).
5. For diagnosis of diffuse pulmonary infections, sometimes associated with Adult Respiratory Distress Syndrome, sometimes in AIDS patients, when less invasive methods have failed (Dijkman et al. 1982; Dijkman 1989; Rodgers 1979).

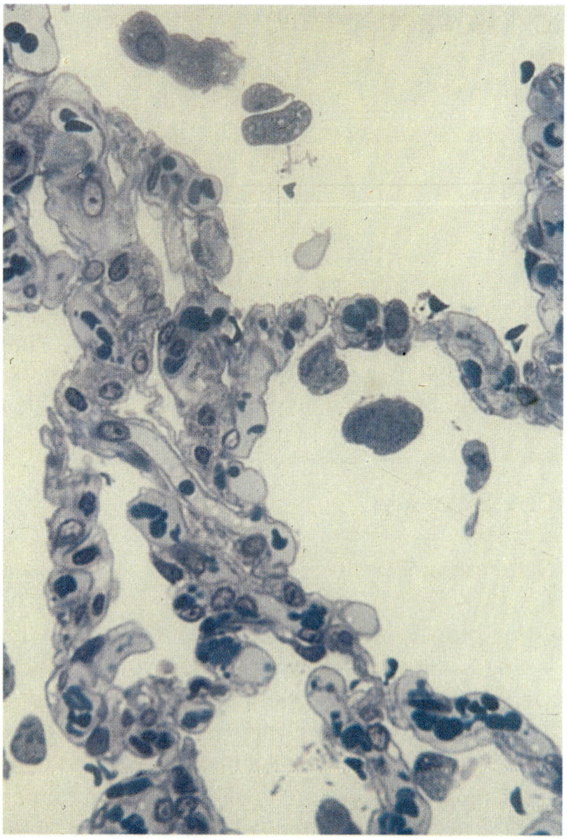

A

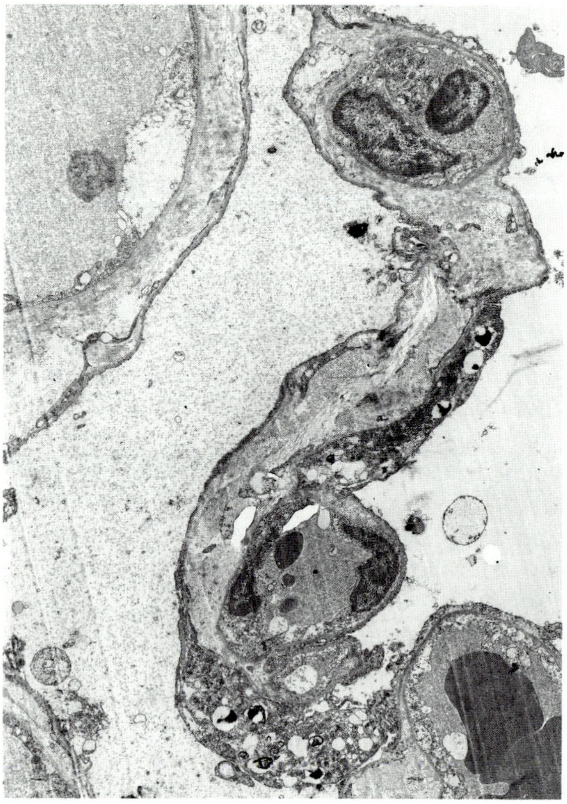

B

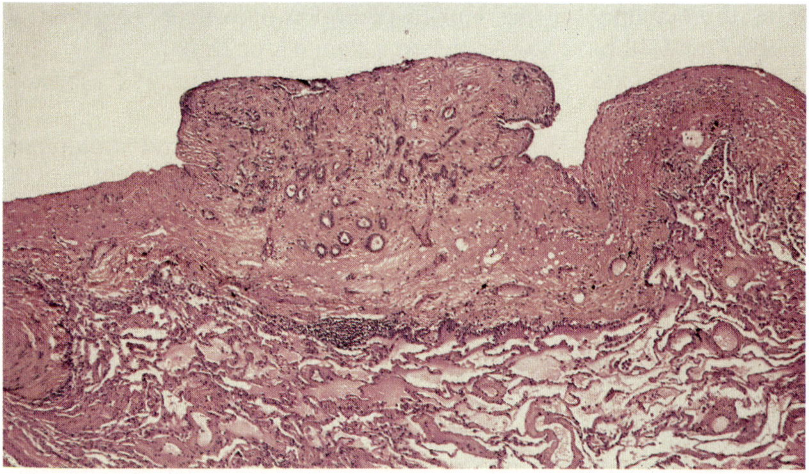

C

Fig. 64 A–C. Pulmonary biopsy using coagulating forceps. Section of normal lung **A** under a light microscope lens, and **B** under an electron microscope. The structure of the parenchyma has been well preserved despite coagulation (see Fig. 30). **C** invasion of the visceral pleura by mesothelioma. Underneath, the lung is normal

Of course, when information is needed on the more central portions of the lung, i.e., the bronchioles or blood vessels, there is no substitute for open surgical biopsy. This is certainly the case in suspected pulmonary vasculitis and in bronchiolitis obliterans.

8.1.2 Contraindications

Contraindications include the absence of a pleural space (spontaneous pleural symphysis), end-stage pulmonary fibrosis with honeycomb lung (the high risk of bronchopleural fistula when biopsying a cystic lung should be remembered), respiratory insufficiency requiring continuous ventilatory support, pulmonary arterial hypertension, and bleeding dyscrasias.

8.1.3 Associated Morbidity

Except for one death no other serious complications were reported in 10 different series covering a total of 1031 patients (Table 11). Water-seal bubbling, indicating an air leak, continued for several days in 2%–5% of the cases reported. In our series, the average length of chest tube drainage was 4 days. Rodgers (1981) performed 86 pulmonary biopsies on children, of which 42 were immunodeficient with suspected opportunistic pneumonias. The complications he reported were more numerous than those in nonimmunodeficient patients: four cases of pneumothorax in patients with *Pneumocystis carinii* infections, where the lung is edematous and inelastic; and two cases of thrombocytopenia and anemia, with bleeding requiring transfusions for 4 days.

Table 11. Thoracoscopic pulmonary biopsy: diagnostic yield and complications

	Diagnostic yield (%)	No of Patients	Hemorrhage	Pneumothorax	Infection	Death
Brandt (1981)	87	467	1	–	–	–
Dijkman (1989)	98	65	1	10	2	1
Faurschou (1985a)	100	7	–	–	–	–
Guy et al. (1983)	100	14	6	3	–	–
Janik et al. (1982)	100	17	–	–	–	–
Kapsenberg (1981)	95	115	–	6	–	–
Rodgers (1981)	94	81	3	4	–	–
Voellmy (1981)	75	32	–	–	–	–
Wetzer et al. (1980)	89	63	–	–	–	–
Boutin (unpublished)	96	170	–	7	1	–
Total	93	1031	5	30	3	1

We performed 170 thoracoscopic lung biopsies, and only once had to send the patient to a surgeon to close a pulmonary breach held open by an adjacent parietal adhesion of the lung.

8.1.4 Results

In our department, large pulmonary samples were taken in every case; with practice, we obtained biopsies with several hundred alveoli that could be analyzed on histologic sections (Fig. 64). A positive diagnosis was made in over 95% of our cases, both with chronic interstitial processes and in peripheral coin lesions or in various localized peripheral pulmonary diseases. We obtained the same percentage of positive diagnoses as Dijkman, using thoracoscopy, and as Wall and Gaensler using thoracotomy (Table 12). This approach, therefore, shows great promise.

We found thoracoscopic pulmonary biopsy to be very useful in the search for asbestos fibers, for a mineralogic study carried out in collaboration with Sebastien (1982) from LEPI and CERCHAR laboratories in Paris. In a group of 25 "control" patients undergoing thoracoscopy for other reasons, who had not been in known contact with asbestos, fiber counts were as follows (Table 13):

$1.4 \pm 0.3 \times 10^6$ chrysotile fibers/g dry tissue, and
$1.0 \pm 0.4 \times 10^6$ amphibole fibers/g dry tissue

These figures strongly contrast with the following values obtained in subjects with known asbestos exposure:

$19.5 \pm 11.5 \times 10^6$ chrysotile fibers/g dry tissue, and
$10.8 \pm 2.6 \times 10^6$ amphibole fibers/g dry tissue

Contrary to the opinion of Churg and Wood (1983), thoracoscopic pulmonary biopsy seems to be an excellent method for sampling the peripheral lung for mineralogic studies.

Table 12. Results of surgical or thoracoscopic pulmonary biopsy in patients who have previously undergone unsuccessful transbronchial biopsy

	Surgery Wall Gaensler (1981)	Thoracoscopy Dijkman (1982a)	Thoracoscopy Boutin (1982a)
No of patients	33	63	39
Diagnoses:			
Sarcoidosis	7	7	4
Histiocytosis	–	5	–
Cancer	–	5	7
Pneumoconiosis	–	7	13
Lymphangiomyomatosis	–	3	1
Diffuse interstitial fibrosis:	13	17	10
· Bronchiolitis	1	–	–
· LIP	–	–	2
· DIP	2	–	2
· UIP	10	–	5
Fibrosis	3	7	1
Granulomatosis	6	3	1
Varia	–	3	1
Undiagnosed	4	–	2
Sensitivity	29/33 = 88%	57/63 = 90.5%	37/39 = 95%

LIP, lymphocytic interstitial pneumonitis; DIP, desquamative interstitial pneumonitis; UIP, usual interstitial pneumonitis

Table 13. Assessment of asbestos burden by thoracoscopic lung biopsy: mean asbestos fiber counts ($\times 10^6$ per gram of dried lung tissue) $\pm$SEM

	Control patients ($n = 25$)	Occupational exposure ($n = 30$)	North Corsican environmental exposure ($n = 8$)
Chrysotile	1.4 ± 0.3	19.5 ± 11.5 (NS)*	2.7 ± 1.5 (NS)*
Amphiboles	1 ± 0.4	10.8 ± 2.6 ($p < .001$)*	20.1 ± 8.1 ($p < .001$)*

Biopsy samples were analyzed by electron microscopy according to Sebastien (1982) technique: pulmonary asbestos burden correlates with known asbestos exposure, whether occupational or environmental (patients from North Corsica)

* Student's *t* test vs mean fiber counts in control (unexposed) patients

8.2 Empyema

Empyema develops in three stages: exudative, fibropurulent, and organizing (Le Roux et al. 1986; Light 1983). According to Le Roux, "in the exudative, early stage, pleural liquid is thin and has a low cellular content, and the visceral pleura and related lung are mobile. In the fibropurulent, transitional stage, large numbers of polymorphonuclear leukocytes have appeared in the liquid and fibrin deposition on both pleural surfaces has begun to limit the extent of the empyema and to immobilize the lung. In the final stage of organization, the liquid content is thick and fibroblasts have invaded the thickened fibrous layers over the visceral and parietal pleurae. These differences have important therapeutic implications."

Relatively Early Cases. In the exudative stage, the pleural fluid is rather thin and can be aspirated easily with a syringe and plastic catheter, or, preferably, with a 3-mm pleural trocar (see p. 13). Within days however, it may become thick and difficult to aspirate with the simple thoracentesis technique. Unless it is a complication of thoracotomy, empyema is nearly always localized posteriorly, sometimes extending to the lateral wall. It frequently presents as a posteriorly situated D-shaped radiographic density on chest roentgenograms. A chest tube is then difficult to insert, painful for the patient and usually unnecessary. Indeed, streptokinase or urokinase instillations and daily pleural lavage achieve good results in most cases.

More Advanced (Fibropurulent) Cases (Figs. 65, 66). As a consequence of both the course of the disease and of previous pleural punctures, X-rays may show multiple loculations, often with air-fluid levels which are difficult to evacuate with simple needle puncture. There is sometimes an associated bronchopleural fistula. Tube thoracostomy should be considered in these patients, according to criteria defined by Light regarding pleural pH, and pleural levels of glucose and lactic dehydrogenase. Generally speaking, the indications for tube insertion become stronger with lower pH, lower glucose levels, and higher levels

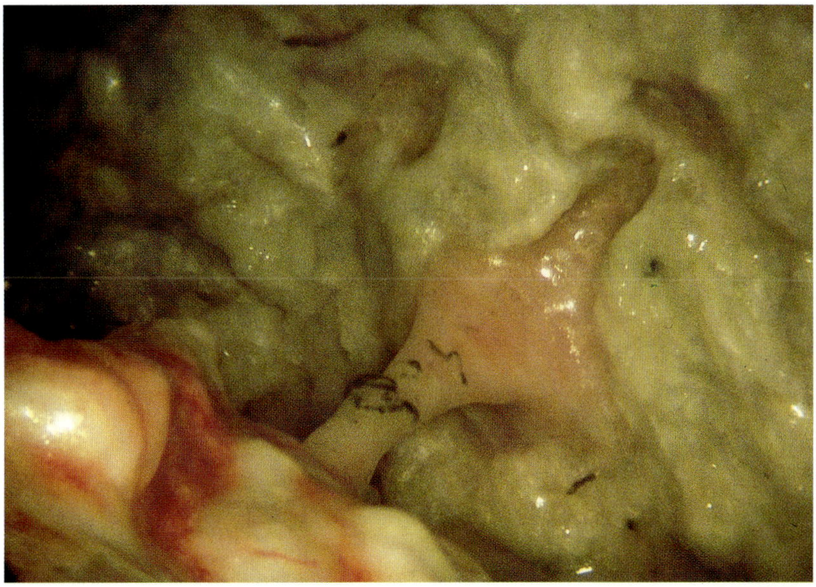

Fig. 65. Empyema: fibropurulent stage. The pleura is completely covered by a greenish, purulent exudate spread evenly over the parietal pleura and the lung, which can be seen in the foreground on the *bottom left*. The patient responded within 4 days of treatment with antibiotics and chest tube drainage, using a long 30 Fr tube placed under direct vision

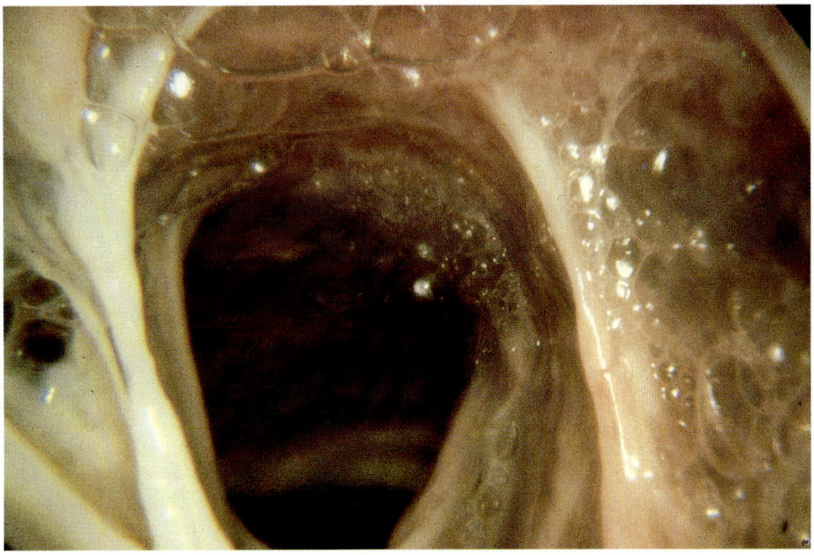

Fig. 66. Multilocular empyema: fibropurulent stage. Adhesions of this type can create partitions with pockets of pus that are impossible to puncture and drain completely, except under visual control. These adhesions and pockets can be broken up with thoracoscopic forceps, resulting in a large, single cavity which can be drained thoroughly, ensuring that the patient recovers quickly with minimal sequellae

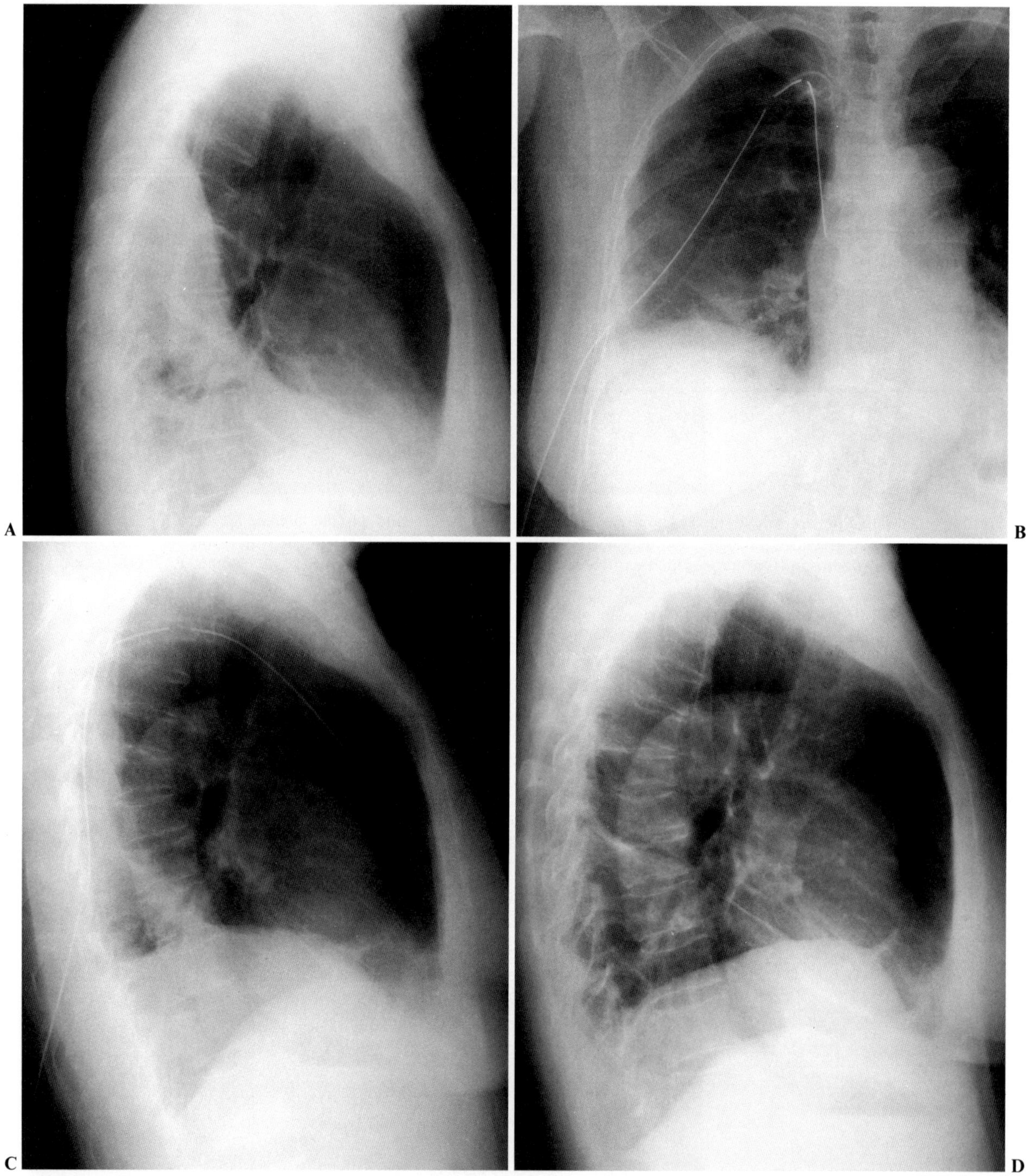

Fig. 67 A–D. Empyema: radiographic findings. **A** A large loculated effusion which could not be drained completely with simple thoracenteses. **B** After thoracoscopic breakup of the partitions, frontal roentgenogram done at the termination of the procedure suggests complete drainage of the purulent fluid. **C** Lateral view confirms excellent pleural drainage. **D** Empyema appears resolved on lateral view taken shortly after chest tube removal 3 days after thoracoscopy

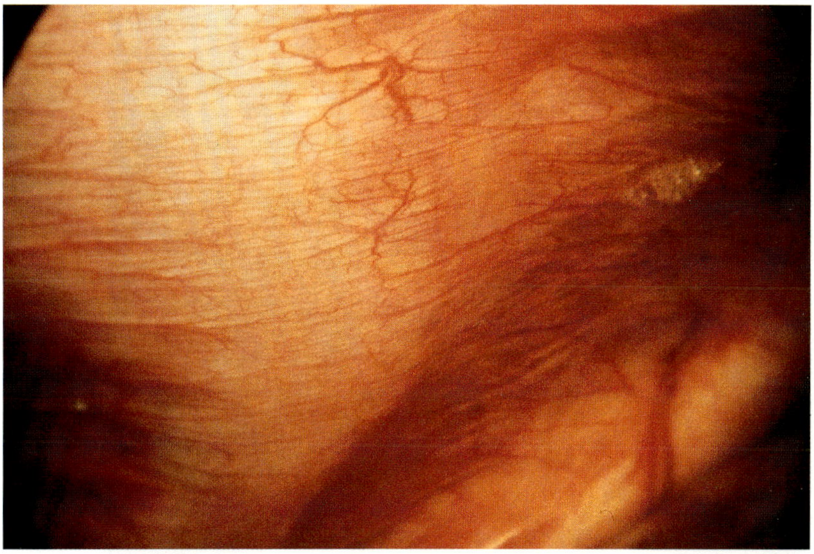

Fig. 68. Parietal pleural tumors. Many parietal pleural tumors can be approached during thoracoscopy: fibromas, lipomas, fibrosarcomas, neurofibromas, diaphragmatic tumors, pleuropericardial cysts, etc. Thoracoscopy provides more precise information and better tissue than percutaneous needle biopsy under CT scan control. The procedure is straightforward: induced pneumothorax is performed on the endoscopy table at the beginning of the procedure, and the lung is promptly reexpanded at the end. The chest tube is removed as soon as roentgenogram confirms that the lung is re-approximated to the chest wall, and the patient can return home a few hours later. All tissue tests can be performed on biopsy material: cytological, histological, electronic microscopy, a mineralogical study, immunofluorescence studies, etc.

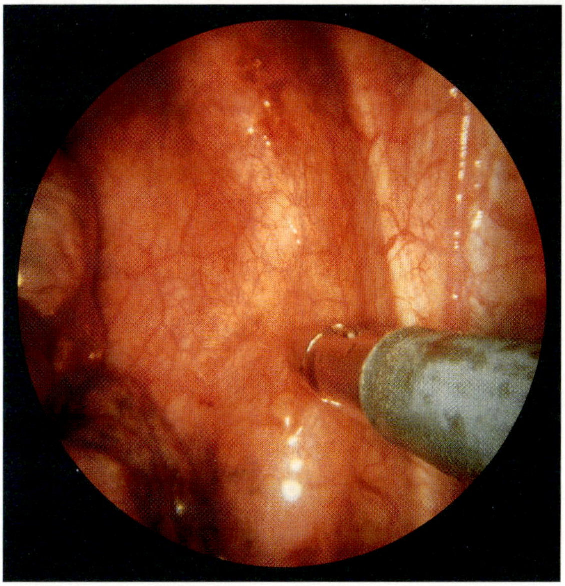

Fig. 69. Mediastino-thoracoscopy. The pericardium can be easily explored. There is no risk involved if biopsies are taken on the left. It is very dangerous to take biopsies on the right (see Sect. 3.6.3). The mediastinal lymph nodes can also be accessed: on the left above the aorta (Fig. 22); on the *right* as shown here. The superior vena cava *(blue, running vertically)* is crossed by the phrenic nerve from top to bottom. In the *back left,* there is the brachiocephalic arterial trunk. In the *background* at 7 and 9 o'clock, parts of the lung can be seen. Here the mediastinal pleura is being opened. Initially, the lymph nodes seen *above* and *below* the forceps in the photo were aspirated for cytologic studies. This also reassures the endoscopist that the structure is not vascular. With this assurance, biopsies of the nodes may also be taken with the cauterizing forceps

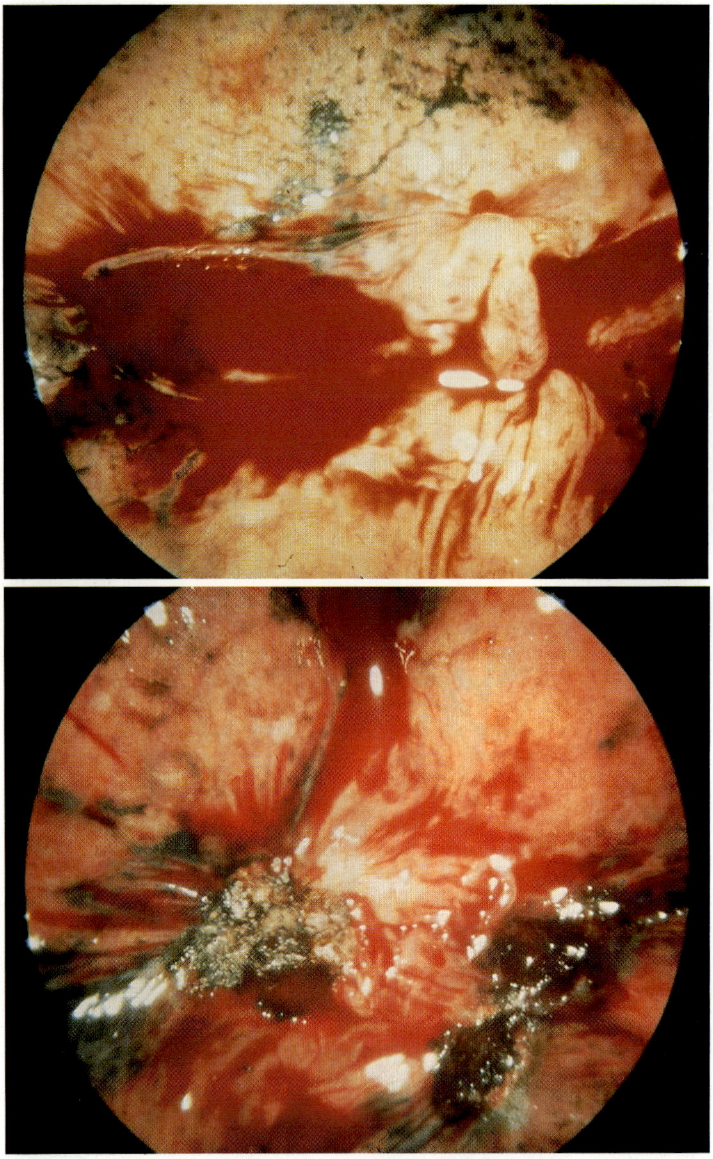

A

B

Fig. 70 A, B. Pulmonary biopsy - laser. **A** When biopsies are taken using simple forceps without coagulation, the YAG laser can be used to coagulate the lung. The opening of two pulmonary biopsies can be seen. **B** With laser output set at 40 W, the pulmonary parenchyma retracts easily, and after 3-5 pulses, the "hole" closes and aerostasis is achieved. Apart from pulmonary biopsy, the laser can be used to control any hemorrhage caused by biopsies of the parietal pleura. It can also coagulate blebs or emphysematous bullae which are less than 2 cm in diameter. The laser can also be used to control hemorrhages due to pleural or pulmonary wounds. Lastly it makes the cutting off of adhesions much easier

of LDH. Light suggests that early tube insertion shortens the time required for treatment when necessary, i.e., when pH <7.00 (and perhaps 7.20), when glucose is <40 mg/100 ml, and when LDH is >1000 Units (Light et al. 1980b; Light 1985).

If chest tube drainage becomes necessary, thoracoscopy helps place the tube under direct vision. In order to break up loculations of pus, the numerous adhesions are severed (Fig. 67), one at a time, using forceps, HF coagulation, or laser, usually without any difficulty. This creates one large, unilocular cavity. A large drainage tube is inserted low in the thorax, under direct vision, and is pushed as high as possible into the dome; the lung is immediately reexpanded.

These steps usually ensure drainage of most thoracic pus within an hour, which eventually will shorten the duration of tube drainage, the course of the disease, and will reduce hospital time.

8.3 Diverse Indications

Unusual circumstances where thoracoscopy has been useful include diagnostic studies for rare parietal pleural tumors (Fig. 68), whether benign or malignant, neurinomas, thymomas and other anterior mediastinal tumors, mediastinal lymph nodes when mediastinoscopy has been unsuccessful (Fig. 69), and transdiaphragmatic hepatic biopsy (Canto 1981).

Therapeutic applications include sympathetic nerve section (J. C. Guerin 1989a; Toomes and Linder 1989), clot removal for postoperative or traumatic hemothorax, pericardial drainage or biopsy, talcage for chylothorax, etc.

New techniques, such as laser coagulation (Fig. 70), are still being perfected. Perhaps a biological glue will eventually replace talc or tetracycline for pleural symphysis. New immunologic drugs such as interferon or interleukin-2 bear great hope for the future.

Today, in well-defined circumstances, thoracoscopy is a safe, effective technique for diagnosis and treatment, available to all pulmonologists who have taken the time to master the procedure. Experience and training are essential to learning all uses of thoracoscopy as well as to know its limitations. In light of its effectiveness, its excellent patient tolerance, along with minimal costs compared with thoracotomy, one can reasonably hope that thoracoscopy will spread widely, to the great benefit of our patients.

References

Abrams LD (1958) A pleural punch biopsy. Lancet 1: 30-31

Adler RH, Rappole BW (1967) Recurrent malignant pleural effusions and talc powder aerosol treatment. Surgery 62: 1000-1006

Aherne T (1982) Thoracoscopy in management of pleural effusions. Irish Med J 75: 406-407

Alcozer G, Dorigoni A (1984) La toracoscopia diagnostica. Nardini, Florence

Alexander J (1937) The collapse therapy of pulmonary tuberculosis. Charles C. Thomas, Springfield, III, 313-316

Almany SL, Sherman S (1987) Tetracycline chemical pleurodesis for spontaneous pneumothorax. Am Rev Respir Dis 135: A421

Almind M, Lange P, Viskum K (1989) Spontaneous pneumothorax: comparison of simple drainage, talc pleurodesis and tetracycline pleurodesis. Thorax 44: 627-630

Anderson CB, Philpott GW, Ferguson TB (1974) The treatment of malignant pleural effusions. Cancer 33: 916-922

Antman KH (1980) Malignant mesothelioma. New Engl J Med 303: 200-202

Antman KH, Aisner J (1987) Asbestos related malignancy. Grune and Stratton, Orlando

Antony VB, Sahn SA, Repine JE (1985a) Experimental models of inflammation in the pleural space. In: Chretien J, Bignon J, Hirsch A (eds) the pleura in health and disease. Dekker, New York, pp 387-400

Antony VB, Owen CL, Sahn SA (1985b) Mechanisms of Tetracycline induced pleural fibrosis: tetracycline stimulates fibroblast proliferation in vivo and in vitro. Am Rev Respir Dis 131: A33

Antony VB (1987) Pleurodesis - testing the waters. Am Rev Respir Dis 135: 775-776

Artvinli M, Sahin AA, Altinors M, Baris YI (1981) Thoracoscopy in the diagnosis of environmental natural mineral fiber-induced pleural diseases. Poumon-Coeur 37: 245-247

Ash SR, Manfredi F (1974) Directed biopsy using a small endoscope: thoracoscopy and peritoneoscopy simplified. New Engl J Med 291: 1398-1399

Audier M, Boutin C, Arnaud A, D'Journo J (1967) A propos d'un cas d'épanchement cardiaque traité par talcage pleuroscopique. Marseille Med 104: 866-869

Austgen M (1989) Palliative Therapie tumorbedingter Pleuraergüsse mit Radioisotopen. Pneumologie 43: 88-91

Austin EH, Flye MW (1979) The treatment of recurrent malignant pleural effusion. Ann Thorac Surg 28: 190-203

Bariffi F, Goatley M, Illiano A, Pezza A, Tranfa CME (1979) Indications thérapeutiques dans le pneumothorax spontané idiopathique. Bronchopneumologie 29: 501-505

Bayle JY, Pirollet B, Guerin JC (1988) Apport de la thoracoscopie dans l'histiocytose X pulmonaire. Rev Pneumol Clin 44: 292-295.

Bayly TC, Kisner DL, Sybert A, Macdonald JS, Tsou E, Schein PS (1978) Tetracycline and Quinacrine in the control of malignant pleural effusions. A randomized trial. Cancer 41: 1188-1192

Beattie EJ (1963) The treatment of malignant pleural effusions by partial pleurectomy. Surg Clin N Am 43: 99-108

Beaulieu M, Despres JP, Lemieux M (1972) Médiastino-pleuroscopie: une nouvelle technique de diagnostic des maladies du thorax. Chirurgie 98: 355-359

Bejui-Thivolet F, Guerin JC, Salle M, Milox A, Champel F, Vitrey D (1984) La thoracoscopie avec brossage pleural. Un nouveau mode diagnostique des affections de la plèvre. Rev Pneumol Clin 40: 311-319

Ben-Isaac FE, Simmons DH (1975) Flexible fiberoptic pleuroscopy: pleural and lung biopsy. Chest 67: 573-576

Benda R, Aubin M (1955) Pneumothorax spontané non tuberculeux. Perforation vérifiée par pleuroscopie. Comportement paradoxal des différents lobes après talcage. J Franç Med Chir Thor 9: 157-159

Bense L (1987) Pathogenetic factors and treatment of spontaneous pneumothorax. Thesis, Stockholm

Bergqvist S, Nordenstam H (1966) Thoracoscopy and pleural biopsy in the diagnosis of pleurisy. Scand J Respir Dis 47: 64-74

Bernhard WF, Malcon JA, Berry RW, Wylie RH (1962) A study of the pathogenesis and management of spontaneous pneumothorax. Dis Chest 41: 403-412

Bethune N (1935) Pleural poudrage. A new technic for the deliberate production of pleural adhesions as a preliminary to lobectomy. J Thorac Cardiovasc Surg 4: 251-261

Blanchette G, Meunier N, Provost G (1973) Ensemencement métastatique par biopsie pleurale. L'Union Med Canada 102: 330-334

Bloomberg AE (1970) Thoracoscopy in diagnosis of pleural effusions. NY State J Med 19: 1974-1977

Bloomberg AE (1978) Thoracoscopy in perspective. Surg Gynecol Obstet 147: 433-443

Boniface E, Guerin JC (1989) Intérêt du talcage par thoracoscopie dans le traitement symptomatique des pleurésies récidivantes. A propos de 302 cas. Rev Mal Resp 6: 133-139

Bonnefoy M, Guerin JC, Kalb JC (1978) Le traitement du pneumothorax (à propos d'une série de 160 cas). Lyon Med 240: 303-306

Bouchama A, Chastre J, Gaudichet A, Soler P, Gibert C (1984) Acute pneumonitis with bilateral pleural effusion after talc pleurodesis. Chest 86: 795-797

Boushy SF, North LB, Helgason AH (1978) Thoracoscopy: technique and results in eighteen patients with pleural effusion. Chest 74: 386-389

Boutin C, Arnaud A, Rocca-Serra JP, Taranger J, Charpin J (1968) Le diagnostic des pleurésies tuberculeuses. Intérêt de la ponction-biopsie de plèvre et de la culture du fragment. Rev Tuberc Pneumol 32: 37-46

Boutin C (1975a) Aspects actuels des pleurésies tuberculeuses. Med Hyg 33: 1365-1369

Boutin C, Arnaud A, Farisse P, Viallat J, Choux R, Aimard A, Belnet M (1975b) Les biopsies pleurales: incidents et rentabilité actuelle de la biopsie à l'aiguille d'Abrams. A propos de 1.000 prélèvements. Intérêt de la biopsie pleuroscopique. Poumon-Coeur 31: 317-321

Boutin C, Cargnino P, Viallat JR (1979) La thoracoscopie: intérêt actuel. Sa place dans le diagnostic des pleurésies chroniques. Poumon-Coeur 35: 23-29

Boutin C, Cargnino P, Viallat JR (1980) Thoracoscopy in the early diagnosis of malignant pleural effusions. Endoscopy 12: 155-160

Boutin C, Viallat JR, Cargnino P, Farisse P (1981a) Thoracoscopy in malignant pleural effusions. Am Rev Respir Dis 124: 588-592

Boutin C, Viallat JR, Cargnino P, Farisse P, Choux R (1981b) La Thoracoscopie en 1980. Revue générale. Poumon-Coeur 37: 11-19

Boutin C, Sebastien P, Janson X, Viallat JR (1981c) Métrologie des fibres minérales dans les biopsies thoracoscopiques pulmonaires et pleurales. Résultats préliminaires. Poumon-coeur 37: 253-257

Boutin C, Viallat JR, Cargnino P, Farisse P (1981d) Indications actuelles de la thoracoscopie. Rev Fr Mal Resp 9: 309-318

Boutin C, Jullian H, Viallat JR, Sebastien P, Cargnino P (1981e). La biopsie pulmonaire par thoracoscopie. Etude préliminaire. Rev Fr Mal Resp 9: 337-344

Boutin C, Viallat JR, Cargnino P, Rey F (1982a) Thoracoscopic lung biopsy. Experimental and clinical preliminary study. Chest 82: 44-48

Boutin C, Cargnino P, Viallat JR, Rey F (1982b) Thoracoscopie. Encycl Med Chir. Poumon, Paris

Boutin C, Irisson M, Rathelot P, Petite JM (1983) L'extension pariétale des mésothéliomes pleuraux malins diffus après biopsies. Prévention par radiothérapie. Presse Med 29: 1823

Boutin C, Farisse P, Rey F, Viallat JR, Cargnino P (1984) La thoracoscopie doit-elle être un examen de routine en pratique pneumologique courante? Med Hyg 42: 2992-3000

Boutin C, Viallat JR, Cargnino P, Farisse P, Irisson M, Rey F, Velardocchio JM (1985a) thoracoscopy. In: Chretien J, Bignon J, Hirsch A (eds) The pleura in health and disease. Dekker, New York, pp 587-622

Boutin C, Rey F, Viallat JR (1985b) Etude randomisée de l'efficacité du talcage thoracoscopique et de l'instillation de tétracycline dans le traitement des pleurésies cancéreuses récidivantes. Rev Mal Resp 2: 374

Boutin C, Viallat JR, Rey F (1986a) A propos du talcage pleural. Presse Med 15: 123

Boutin C (1986b) The laser in thoracoscopy. Tumor Diagnos Ther 7: 33-35

Boutin C, Viallat JR, Rey F (1986c) Thoracoscopy in diagnosis, prognosis and treatment of mesothelioma. In: Antman K, Aisner J (eds) Asbestos related malignancy. Grune and Straton, New York, pp. 301-321

Boutin C, Rey F, Viallat JR (1988a) Aspects diagnostiques du mésothéliome malin de la plèvre. Rev Mal Resp 5: R28

Boutin C, Mathlouthi A, Espinasse P, Viallat JR, Rey F, Fincker F, Pasquier J (1988b) Perméabilité alvéolaire au cours des épanchements et après symphyse pleurale au talc. Rev Fr Mal Resp 5, Sup 1: R125

Boutin C (1989a) The laser in thoracoscopy. Pneumologie 43: 96-97

Boutin C (1989b) Thoracoscopy in malignant mesothelioma. Pneumologie 43: 61-65

Boutin C (1989c) La symphyse pleurale par talcage sous thoracoscopie. Rev Mal Resp 6: 91-93

Boutin C, Viallat JR, Rey F, Astoul P, Seitz B (1989d). Thoracoscopy in malignant mesothelioma. Chest 96: 275 S

Brandt HJ, Mai J (1971) Differentialdiagnose des Pleuraergusses durch Thorakoskop. Pneumologie 145: 192-203

Brandt HJ (1974) Diagnostik der Pleuraerkrankungen einschließlich Thorakoskopie und Biopsie. Thoraxchirurgie 22: 371-380

Brandt HJ (1977) Endoskopie und Biopsie in der Diagnostik pneumologischer Krankheiten. Prax Pneumol 31: 384-401

Brandt HJ (1978) Indikation und Technik der diagnostischen Thorakoskopie. Atemwegs Lungenkrankh 3: 150-160

Brandt HJ (1981) Biopsie pulmonaire sous contrôle visuel. Poumon-Coeur 37: 307-311

Brandt HJ, Loddenkemper R, Mai J (1985) Atlas of diagnostic thoracoscopy. Thieme, Stuttgart

Brenner J, Sordillo PP, Magill GB, Golbey RB (1982) Malignant mesothelioma of the pleura. Review of 123 patients. Cancer 49: 2431-2435

Brinkman GL (1959) The significance of pleural effusion complicating otherwise operable bronchogenic carcinoma. Dis Chest 36: 152-154

Brocard H, Brincourt J, Thenot A (1961) L'étiologie des pneumothorax spontanés actuellement observés. Bull Mém Soc Méd Hop 56: 803-815

Buchwald J (1984) Fibrinklebung beim Pneumothorax und in der langen Parechymchirurgie. In: Scheele J (ed) Fibrinklebung. Springer, Berlin Heidelberg New York, pp 169-172

Butchart EG, Ashcroft T, Barnsley WC, Holden MP (1976) Pleuropneumonectomy in the management of diffuse malignant mesothelioma of the pleura. Experience with 29 patients. Thorax 31: 15-24

Canto A, Blasco E, Casillas M, Zarza AG, Padilla J, Pastor J, Tarazona V, Paris F (1977) Thoracoscopy in the diagnosis of pleural effusion. Thorax 32: 550-554

Canto A (1981a) Thoracoscopie: résultats dans les cancers de la plèvre. Poumon-Coeur 37: 235-239

Canto A, Paris F, Rivas J, Ferrer G, Moya J, Borro J, Morera R (1981b) Toracoscopia ampliada a la exploracion del espacio subfrenico. Tecnica original. Rev Esp Cirg CTV 2: 514-518

Canto A, Rivas J, Saumench J, Morera R, Moya J (1983) Points to consider when choosing a biopsy method in cases of pleurisy of unknown origin. Chest 84: 176-179

Canto A, Rivas J, Moya J, Saumench J, Pac J, Morera R, Ferrer G (1985a) Pleural effusion of malignant etiology. Thoracoscopic use of talc as an effective method of pleurodesis. Med Clin 84: 806-808

Canto A, Ferrer G, Romagosa V, Moya J, Bernat R (1985b) Lung cancer and pleural effusion. Clinical significance and study of pleural metastatic locations. Chest 87: 649-352

Canto A (1989) Diagnostic results in secondary malignant pleural effusions. Pneumologie 43: 58-60

Chahinian AP (1983) Therapeutic Modalities in Malignant Pleural Mesothelioma. In: Chretien J, Hirsch A (eds) Diseases of the pleura. Masson, New York, pp 224-236

Chahinian PA (1985) Management of pleural tumors and malignant pleural effusions. In: Chretien J, Bignon J, Hirsch A (eds) The pleura in health and disease. Dekker, New York, pp 571-584

Chambers JS (1958) Palliative treatment of neoplastic pleural effusion with intercostal intubation and talc instillation. West J Surg Obstet Gynecol 26-28

Chretien J, Andre-Bougaran J (1967) La ponction-biopsie de la plèvre pariétale à l'aiguille dans le diagnostic étiologique des épanchements pleuraux. Etude de 847 prélèvements. Soc Med Hop, Paris 118: 1143-1154

Chretien J, Hirsch A (eds) (1983) Diseases of the pleura. Masson, New York

Chretien J, Bignon J, Hirsch A (eds) (1985) The pleura in health and disease. Dekker, New York

Churg A, Warnock ML, Bensch KG (1978) Malignant mesothelioma arising after direct application of asbestos and fiber glass to the pericardium. Am Rev Respir Dis 118: 419-424

Churg A, Wood P (1983) Observations on the distribution of asbestos fibers in human lungs. Environ Res 31: 374-380

Collins TR, Sahn SA (1987) Thoracocentesis. Clinical value, complications, technical problems, and patient experience. Chest 91: 817-822

Cope C (1958) A New pleural biopsy needle-preliminary study. JAMA 167: 1107-1108

Coulaud E, Deschamps, P (1947) Découverte pleuroscopique d'une importante perforation pulmonaire asymptomatique. Guérison rapide spontanée. Rev Tuberculose 11: 825-827

Cova F (1927) Thoracoscopia - operazione di Jacobaeus. Sperling and Kupper, Milan

Cova F (1928) Atlas thoracoscopicon. 1er Atlas dessiné. Sperling and Kupper, Milan

Davidoff D, Naparstek Y, Eliakim M (1983) The use of pleurodesis for intractable pleural effusion due to congestive heart failure. Postgrad Med J 59: 330-331

Davidson AC, George RJ, Sheldon CD, Sinha G, Corrin B, Geddes DM (1988) Thoracoscopy: assessment of a physician service and comparison of a flexible bronchoscope used as a thoracoscope with a rigid thoracoscope. Thorax 43: 327-332

De Camp PT, Moseley PW, Scott ML, Hatch HB JR (1973) Diagnostic thoracoscopy. Ann Thorac Surg 16: 79-84

Decker DA, Dines DE, Payne WS, Bernatz PE, Pairolero PC (1978) The significance of a cytologically negative pleural effusion in bronchogenic carcinoma. Chest 74: 640-642

Deslauriers J, Beaulieu M, Dufour C, Michaud P, Despres JP, Lemieux M (1976) Mediastinopleuroscopy: a new approach to the diagnosis of intrathoracic diseases. Ann Thorac Surg 22: 265-269

Dijkman JH, Van der Meer JW, Bakker W, Wever AM, Van der Broek PJ (1982) Transpleural lung biopsy by the thoracoscopic route in patients with diffuse interstitial pulmonary disease. Chest 82: 76-83

Dijkman JH (1989) Thorakoskopie bei immunsupprimierten Patienten. Pneumologie 43: 116-118

Dines DE, Pierre RV, Franzen SJ (1975) The value of cells in the pleural fluid in the differential diagnosis. Mayo Clin Proc 50: 571-572

Douady D, Meyer A (1942) Manuel de pleuroscopie et de section de brides dans le pneumothorax thérapeutique. Legrand A and Bertrand J, Paris

Driscoll PJ, Aronstam EM (1961) Experiences in the management of recurrent spontaneous pneumothorax. J Thorac Cardiovasc Surg 42: 174-178

Dumarest F (1914) Cinq ans de pratique du pneumothorax artificiel. Résultats. Bull Med Paris 28: 15-18

Dumarest J, Galy P, Germain J (1954) La pratique du pneumothorax thérapeutique. Masson, Paris

Dunkel TB (1986) Intrapleural Tetracycline in the treatment of malignant pleural effusions. Minnesota Med 69: 717-725

Elert O, Eigel P (1986) Treatment of idiopathic spontaneous pneumothorax; transthoracic endoscopic use of fibrine glue. In: Schlag G, Redl H (eds) Fibrin sealant in operative medicine. Springer, Berlin Heidelberg New York, vol 5, pp 107-114

Elmes PC, Simpson MJC (1976) The clinical aspects of mesothelioma. Q J Med 179: 427-449

Escamilla R, Meresse C, Sallerin F, Hermant C, Krempf M, Migueres J (1986) Intérêt du talcage de plèvre sous pleuroscopie (TPP) dans le traitement des pleurésies malignes. A propos de 101 cas. Bull Eur Physio Resp 22: 79S

Eschapasse H, Fabre J, Toffa R, Hassani M, Gaillard J, Dahan M, Fournial G, Berthoumieu F (1977) Le traitement du pneumothorax spontané à propos d'une série de 88 cas opérés et d'une étude expérimentale chez l'animal. Bronchopneumologie 27: 427-437

Faurschou P (1974) Rheumatoid pleuritis and thoracoscopy. Scand J Resp. Dis 55: 277-283

Faurschou P (1985a) Diagnostic thoracoscopy in pleuro-pulmonary infiltrates without pleural effusion. Endoscopy 17: 21-25

Faurschou P, Francis D, Faarup P (1985b) Thoracoscopic, histological, and clinical findings in nine case of rheumatoid pleural effusion. Thorax 40: 371-375

Faurschou P (1989) Thoracoscopy in rheumatoid pleural effusion. Pneumologie 43: 69-71

Fentiman IS, Millis R, Sexton S, Hayward JL (1981) Pleural effusions in breast cancer. A review of 105 cases. Cancer 47: 2087

Fentiman IS, Rubens RD, Hayward JL (1983) Control of pleural effusions in patients with breast cancer. A randomized trial. Cancer 52: 737-739

Fentiman IS, Rubens RD, Hayward JL (1986) A comparison of intracavitary talc and tetracycline for the control of pleural effusions secondary to breast cancer. Eur J Cancer Clin Oncol 22: 1079-1081

Fentiman IS (1987) Diagnosis and treatment of malignant pleural effusions. Cancer Treat Rev 14: 107-118

Fleishman SJ, Lichter AI, Buchanan G, Sichel RJS (1956) Investigation of idiopathic pleural effusions by thoracoscopy. Thorax 11: 324-327

Forlanini C (1882) A contribuzione della terapia chirurgica nella tisi del polmone: ablazione del polmone? Pneumotorax artificiale ? Gazzetta degli Ospedali 3: 537

Fourestier M, Duret M (1943) Nécessité de la biopsie pleurale pour le diagnostic de l'endothéliome de la plèvre. Presse Med 32: 467-468

Fracchia AA, Knapper WH, Carey JT, Farrow JH (1970) Intrapleural chemotherapy for effusion from metastatic breast carcinoma. Cancer 20: 626-629

Frank W, Grober H, Mai J, Loddenkemper R (1989) Pleurodese mit Tetracyclin-Hydrochlorid. Pneumologie 43: 80-84

Frankel A, Krasna I, Baronofsky ID (1961) An experimental study of pleural symphysis. J Thorac Cardiovasc Surg 42: 43-51

Gaensler EA (1956) Parietal pleurectomy for recurrent spontaneous pneumothorax. Surg Gynecol Obst 102: 293-308

Gaensler EA, Moister MVB, Hamm J (1964) Open-lung biopsy in diffuse pulmonary disease. N Eng J Med 270: 1319-1331

Gamondes JP, Robin J, Maret G (1984) Le traitement chirurgical du pneumothorax spontané par pleurectomie pariétale apicale et voie axillaire. Lyon Chir 80: 306-307

Gernez-Rieux CH, Macquet V, Voisin C, Wattel F, Wallaert C (1966). Pleuroscopie (Cimématographie endopleurale). Film Pierre Gaillard, Filmothèque Pfizer-Clin

Getz SB, Beasley WE (1983) Spontaneous pneumothorax. Am J Surg 145: 823-828

Givel JC, Steinhauslin C, Leuebenger P, Besson A (1984) Pneumothorax spontané: étude d'un collectif médico-chirurgical. Med Hyg 42: 2682-2688

Gobbel VG, Rhea WG, Nelson IA, Daniel RA (1963) Spontaneous pneumothorax. J Thorac Cardiovasc Surg 46: 331-345

Good JT, Sahn SA (1978a) Intrapleural therapy with tetracycline in malignant pleural effusions. The importance of proper technique. Chest 74: 602

Good JT, Taryle DA, Hyers TM, Sahn SA (1978b) Clotting and Fibrinolytic activity of pleural fluid in a Model of pleural adhesions. Am Rev Respir Dis 118: 903-908

Graham GG, Mcdonald JR, Glagett OT, Schmidt HW (1953) Examination of pleural fluid for carcinoma cells. J Thorac Surg 25: 366-370

Gravelyn TR, Michelson MK, Gross BH, Sitrin RG (1987) Tetracycline pleurodesis for malignant pleural effusions. A 10-Year retrospective study. Cancer 59: 1973-1977

Greenwald DW, Philips C, Bennett JM (1978) Management of malignant pleural effusion. J Surg Oncol 10: 361-368

Greschuchna D (1989) Thorakoskopie bei Brustwandprozessen. Pneumologie 43: 119-121

Griffiths MH, Riddell RJ, Xipell JM (1980) Malignant mesothelioma: a review of 35 cases with diagnosis and prognosis. Pathol 12: 591-603

Grosser H, Mai J, Loddenkemper R (1989) Pleurodese mit Tetracyclin-Hydrochlorid beim spontan-pneumothorax. Pneumologie 43: 98-100

Guérin JC, Martinat Y, Champel F, Berger C (1985a) Oblitération d'une fistule broncho-pleurale par laser YAG sous thoracoscopie. Presse Med 14: 1245-1246

Guérin JC, Champel F, Biron E, Kalb JC (1985b) Talcage pleural par thoracoscopie dans le traitement du pneumothorax. Etude d'une série de 109 cas traités en 3 ans. Rev. Mal. Resp 2: 25-29

Guérin JC, Champel F, Martinat Y, Boniface E (1987) Etude thoracoscopique de 6 cas de pneumothorax cataménial. Rev Mal Resp 4: 167-171

Guérin JC, Vanderschueren RG, Boutin C (1987) Pleurodesis with fibrin sealant application during thoracoscopy in the treatment of patients with spontaneous pneumothorax. 6th Congrèss SEP, Amsterdam, abstract 614

Guérin JC, Demolombe S, Brudon JR (1989a) Sympatholyse thoracique par thoracoscopie. A propos de 15 cas. Rev Mal Resp 6: R141

Guérin JC, Van Derschueren RGJRA (1989b) Traitement des pneumothorax récidivants par application de colle de fibrine sous endoscopie. Rev Mal Resp 6: 443-445

Guibert B, Mulsant P, Rolet JP, Latarjet M (1984) Traitement chirurgical du pneumothorax 362 cas. Lyon Chir 80: 307-309

Gunnels JJ (1978) Perplexing pleural effusion. Chest 74: 390-393

Gupta N, Opfell RW, Padova J, Margileth D, Souadjian J (1980) Intrapleural Bleomycin vs. Tetracycline for control of malignant pleural effusion. A randomized study. Proc Am Soc Clin Oncol 21: 366

Gust R, Fabel H (1989) Fibrinkleber-pleurodese bei rezidivierenden malignen pleuraergüssen. Pneumologie 43: 85-87

Guy P, Kasparian P, Guibout P (1983) Biopsies pulmonaires par thoracoscopie. Poumon-Coeur 39: 179-181

Gwin E, Pierce G, Boggan M, Kerby G, Ruth W (1975) Pleuroscopy and pleural biopsy with the flexible fiberoptic bronchoscope. Chest 67: 527-531

Harbecke RG (1980) Intrapleurally given Tetracycline with Lidocaine. JAMA 244: 1899-1900

Harley HRS (1979) Malignant pleural effusions and their treatment by intercostal talc pleurodesis. Br J Dis. Chest 73: 173-177

Hatch HB, Blalock JB (1966) Surgical biopsy of the lung. Surg Clin North Am 46: 1399-1403

Haupt GJ, Camishion RC, Templeton JY, Gibbon JH (1960) Treatment of malignant pleural effusions by talc poudrage. Jama 172: 918-921

Hausheer FH, Yarbro JW (1985) Diagnosis and treatment of malignant pleural effusion. Sem Oncol 12: 54-75

Heimlich HJ (1983) Heimlich valve for chest drainage. Med Instrum 17: 29-31

Heindl W, Pridun N (1986) Endoscopic fibrin pleurodesis in complicated PNO In: Schlag G, Redl H (eds) Fibrin sealant in operative medicine. Springer Verlag, Berlin Heidelberg New York, vol 5, pp 89-93

Heine F (1957) Die Probeexcision aus Veränderungen im Thoraxraum und Lunge unter thorakoskopischer Sicht. Beitr Klin Tub 116: 615-627

Herbert A, Gallagher PJ (1982) Pleural biopsy in the diagnosis of malignant mesothelioma. Thorax 37: 816-821

Hillerdal G, Kiviloog J, Nou E, Steinholtz L (1986) Corynebacterium parvum in malignant pleural effusion. A randomized prospective study. Eur J Respir Dis 69: 204-206

Hirsch A, Brochard P, De Cremoux H, Erkan L, Sebastien P, Di Menza L, Bignon J (1982) Features of asbestos-exposed and unexposed mesothelioma. Am J Ind Med 3: 413-422

Huguenin-Dumittan S, Dottrens A (1981) Résultats de la biopsie à l'aiguille. Poumon-Coeur 37: 35-50

Hunninghake GW, Hemken C, Brady M, Monick M (1986) Immune Interferon is a growth factor for human lung fibroblasts. Am Rev Respir Dis 134: 1025-1028

Hyde L (1963) Spontaneous pneumothorax. Dis Chest 43: 476-480

IARC (1987) Silica and some silicates. Monographs on the evaluation of the carcinogenic risk of chemicals to humans, vol. 42 IARC, Lyon

Jacobaeus HC (1910) Über die Möglichkeit, die Zystoskopie bei Untersuchung seröser Höhlungen anzuwenden. Münch Med Wschr 40: 2090-2092

Jacobaeus HC (1925) Die Thorakoskopie und ihre praktische Bedeutung. Ergebn Ges Med 7: 112-166

Janik JS, Nagaraj HS, Groff DB (1982) Thoracoscopic evaluation of intrathoracic lesions in children. J Thorac Cardiovasc Surg 83: 408-413

Jensik R, Cagle JE, Milloy F, Perlia C, Taylor S, Kofman S, Beattie EJ (1963) Pleurectomy in the treatment of pleural effusion due to metastatic malignancy. J Thorac Cardiovasc Surg 46: 322-330

Jereb B, US-Krasovec M, Cervek J, Soos E (1987) Intrapleural application of human leukocyte Interferon (HLI) in breast cancer patients with ipsilateral pleural carcinomatosis. J Interferon Res 7: 357-363

Johnston WW (1985) The malignant pleural effusion. A review of cytopathologic diagnoses of 584 specimens from 472 consecutive patients. Cancer 56: 905-909

Jones GR (1969) Treatment of recurrent malignant pleural effusion by iodized talc pleurodesis. Thorax 24: 69-73

Kaine JL (1985) Refractory massive pleural effusion in systemic lupus erythematosus treated with talc poudrage. Ann Rheum Dis 44: 61-64

Kaiser D, Wolfart W (1983) Therapeutische Prinzipien zur Behandlung des Spontanpneumothorax unter besonderer Berücksichtigung der thorakoskopischen Emphysemblasenabtragung und Fibrinklebung. Prax Klin Pneumol 37: 979-982

Kaiser D (1989a) The use of fibrin adhesive in relapsing spontaneous pneumothorax. Pneumologie 43: 101-104

Kaiser D (1989b) Indikation zur thorakoskopie beim pleuraempyem. Pneumologie 43: 76-79

Kaiser D (1989c) Fibrinklebung beim spontanpneumothorax. Pneumologie 43: 101-104

Kaiser LR (1987) Diagnostic and therapeutic uses of pleuroscopy (thoracoscopy) in lung cancer. Surg Clin North Am 67: 1081-1086

Kampmeier OF (1928) Concerning certain mesothelial thickenings and vascular plexuses of the mediastinal pleura associated with histiocyte and fat-cell production in the human new born. Anat Rec 39: 201-214

Kapsenberg PD (1981) Thoracoscopic biopsy under visual control. Poumon-Coeur 37: 313-316

Kerby GR, Pierce G, Ruth WE (1975) Clinical experience with pleuroscopy utilizing the bronchofiberscope. Ann ORL 84: 602-606

Kessinger A, Wigton RS (1987) Intracavitary Bleomycin and Tetracycline in the management of malignant pleural effusions: a randomized study. J Surg Oncol 36: 81-83

Knowles JH, Gorlin R, Storey CF (1957) Effects of pleural talc poudrage on pulmonary function. J Thoracic Surg 34: 250-256

Krasnik M, Christensen B, Halkier E, Hoier-Madsen K, Jelnes R, Wied U (1987) Pleurodesis in spontaneous pneumothorax by means of tetracycline. Follow-up evaluation of a method. Scand J Thoracic Cardiovasc Surg 21: 181-182

Kreuser ED, Seifried E, Harsch U, Brass B, Schereml W, Heimpel H (1985) Fibrinpleurodese bei malignen Pleuraergüssen. Dtsch Med Wschr 110: 1365-1368

Ladjimi S, M'Raihi L, Djemel A, Mathlouti A, Ben Ayad F, Segaya M (1989) Resultats du talcage pleural sous thoracoscopie au cours des pleurésies néoplasiques. Rev Mal Resp 6: 147-150.

Lageze P, Galy P, Touraine R, Tissor P, Taine R (1960) Le diagnostic positif des pleurésies cancéreuses isolées cliniquement primitives (A propos de 25 observations). Valeur de la cytologie pleurale et de la biopsie sous pleuroscopie. Rev Lyon med 9: 233-252

Lallemand M, Humbert P (1963) Considérations sur 90 cas de pneumothorax spontané non tuberculeux. Marseille Med 9: 719-725

Lange P, Mortensen J, Groth S (1988) Lung function 22-35 years after treatment of idiopathic spontaneous pneumothorax with talc poudrage or simple drainage. Thorax 43: 559-561

Law MR, Ward FG, Hodson ME, Heard BE (1983) Evidence for longer survival of patients with pleural mesothelioma without asbestos exposure. Thorax 38: 744-746

Law MR, Hodson ME, Turner-Warwick M (1984) Malignant mesothelioma of the pleura: clinical aspects and symptomatic treatment. Eur J Resp Dis 65: 162-168

Leahy BC, Honeybourne D, Brear SG, Carroll KB, Thatcher N, Stretton TB (1985) Treatment of malignant pleural effusions with intrapleural Corynebacterium parvum or Tetracycline. Eur J Respir Dis 66: 50-54

Leff A, Hopewell PC, Costello J (1978) Pleural effusion from malignancy. Ann Intern Med 88: 532-537

Legha SS and Muggia FM (1977) Pleural mesothelioma: clinical features and therapeutic implications. Ann Intern Med 87: 613-621.

Lelong JP, Meyer L (1938) La pleuroscopie comme moyen de diagnostic de diverses affections associées à la tuberculose pulmonaire. Rev Tuberc 4: 917-921

Leophonte P, Basset MF, Pincemin J, Louis A, Fernet P, Delaude A (1983) Mortalité des travailleurs du talc en France. Rev Fr Mal Resp 11: 489-490

Le Roux BT, Mohlala ML, Odell JA, Whitton ID (1986) Suppurative diseases of the lung and pleural space. Part I: Empyema thoracis and lung abscess. Curr Probl Surg 23: 1-89

Le Tacon J (1981) La pleuroscopie. Rappel historique. Poumon-Coeur 37: 5-6

Levine MN, Young JE, Ryan ED, Newhouse MT (1986) Pleural effusion in breast cancer. Thoracoscopy for hormone receptor determination. Cancer 57: 324-327

Lewis RJ, Kunderman PJ, Sisler GE, Mackenzie JW (1976) Direct diagnostic thoracoscopy. Ann Thorac Surg 21: 536-539

Lewis RJ, Sisler GE, Mackenzie JW (1981) Diffuse, mixed malignant pleural mesothelioma. Ann Thorac Surg 31: 53-60

Light RW, Erozan YS, Ball WC (1973) Cells in pleural fluid: their value in differential diagnosis. Arch Intern Med 132: 854-860

Light RW, Ball WC (1973) Glucose and amylase in pleural effusions. JAMA 225: 257-260

Light RW, Jenkinson SG, VU-Dinh Minh, George RB (1980a) Observations on pleural fluid pressures as fluid is withdrawn during thoracentesis. Am Rev Respir Dis 121: 799-804

Light RW, Girard WM, Jenkinson SG, George RB (1980b) Parapneumonic Effusions. Am J Med 69: 507-512

Light RW (1983) Pleural diseases. Lea and Febiger, Philadelphia

Light RW (1985) Management of pleural effusions. In: Chretien J, Bignon J, Hirsch A (eds) The pleura in health and disease. Dekker, New York, pp 789-809

Light RW, Stansbury DW, Brown SE (1986) The Relationship between Pleural Pressures and Changes in Pulmonary Function after Therapeutic Thoracentesis. Am Rev Respir Dis 133: 658-661

Lilienthal H (1922) Letter to the editor. Surg Gynec Obstet 35: 123-124

Lloyd MS (1953) Thoracoscopy and biopsy in the diagnosis of pleurisy with effusion. Q Bull Sea View Hosp 14: 128-133

Loddenkemper R, Mai J, Scheffler N, Brandt HJ (1978a) Prospective individual comparison of blind needle biopsy and of thoracoscopy in the diagnosis and differential diagnosis of tuberculous pleurisy. Scand J Respir Dis Suppl 102: 196-198

Loddenkemper R, Mai J, Scheffler N, Brandt HJ (1978b) Diagnostic yield of blind needle biopsy and of thoracoscopy in pleural effusion - an intraindividual comparison. Endoscopy 10: 143

Loddenkemper R, Mai J, Scheffler N, Brandt HJ (1978c) Wertigkeit bioptischer Verfahren beim Pleuraerguß: Individueller Vergleich zwischen Exsudatuntersuchung, Stanzenbiopsie und Thorakoskopie. Prax Pneumol 32: 334-343

Loddenkemper R (1981) Thoracoscopy: results in non cancerous and idiopathic pleural effusions. Poumon-Coeur 37: 261-264

Loddenkemper R, Engel J, Fabel H, Konietzko N, Magnussen H (1982). Diagnostisches Vorgehen beim Pleuraerguß. Prax Klin Pneumol 36: 447-449

Loddenkemper R (1989) Thorakoskopie-Symposium 1987 - Einführung. Pneumologie 43: 45

Lorch DG (1988) Effect of patient positioning on distribution of Tetracycline in the pleural space during pleurodesis. Chest 93: 527-529

Lynn RB (1965) Spontaneous pneumothorax. Dis Chest 48: 251-254

Maassen W (1972) Direkte thorakoskopie ohne vorherige oder mögliche pneumothoraxanlage. Endoscopie 4: 95-98

Maassen W (1975) Über die Entwicklung der endoskopischen und bioptischen Methode in der Thoraxdiagnostik. Prax Pneumol 29: 716-722

Maassen W (1981) Thoracoscopie et biopsie pulmonaire sans pneumothorax initial. Poumon-Coeur 37: 317-320

Maassen W (1989) Thorakoskopie: chirurgische technik. Pneumologie 43: 53-54

Mai J, Loddenkemper R, Brandt HJ (1989) Diagnostische thorakoskopie bei mediastinalen raumforderungen. Pneumologie 43: 122-125

Marrangoni AG, Storey CF, Geib PO (1955) The management of spontaneous pneumothorax. Am Rev Tuberc 72: 257-267

Martensson G (1981) Thoracoscopy in the diagnosis of malignant mesothelioma. Poumon-Coeur 37: 249-251

Martensson G, Hagmar B, Zettergren L (1984) Diagnosis and prognosis in malignant pleural mesothelioma: a prospective study. Eur J Resp Dis 65: 169-178

Martensson G, Pettersson K, Thiringer G (1985) Differentiation between malignant and non-malignant pleural effusion. Eur J Resp Dis 67: 326-334

Martensson G (1989) Prediction of the diagnostic utility of thoracoscopy in pleural effusion. Pneumologie 43: 72-75

Martigne C, Dumas PJ, Pinoche C, Morales F, Couraud L (1980) Le traitement chirurgical du pneumothorax spontané (analyse d'une série de 93 interventions). Bordeaux Med 13: 1509-1512

Matzel W (1985) Biochemical and cytological features of diffuse mesotheliomas of the pleura. Arch Geschwulstforsch 55: 259-264

Maurel A, Saint Florent G, Vanetti A, Brocard M, Mathey J (1971). Comment traiter un pneumothorax spontané dit "idiopathique" du sujet jeune. Presse Med 79: 283-286

Mc Leod DT, Calverley PMA, Millar JW, Horne NW (1985) Further experience of Corynebacterium parvum in malignant pleural effusion. Thorax 40: 515-518

Mc Loud TC, Isler R, Head J (1980) The radiologic appearance of chemical pleurodesis. Radiology 135: 313-317

Meade RH, Blades BB (1949) The surgical treatment of recurrent and chronic spontaneous pneumothorax of nontuberculous origin. Am Rev Tuberc 60: 683-698

Mejer J, Mortensen KM, Hansen HH (1977) Mepacrine hydrochloride in the treatment of malignant pleural effusion: a controlled randomized trial. Scand J Resp Dis 58: 319-323

Melton LJ, Hepper NG, Offord KP (1979) Incidence of spontaneous pneumothorax in Olmsted County, Minnesota: 1950 to 1974. Am Rev Respir Dis 120: 1379-1382

Mestitz P, Purves MJ, Pollard AC (1958) Pleural biopsy in the diagnosis of pleural effusion. A report of 200 cases. Lancet 1349-1353

Miech G, Stoebner J, Razafindrazaka, Witz JP (1967) Les risques de la ponction biopsie transpariétale. L'inoculation néoplasique (à propos de 2 cas). Presse Med 75: 2803-2806

Migueres J, Jover A, Cantegril A, Girard JJ (1974) Intérêt de la ponction biopsie pleurale à l'aiguille dans le diagnostic des pleurésies non purulentes (A propos de 250 épanchements). Rev Med Toulouse 10: 387

Migueres J, Jover A (1975a) Pleurésies sérofibrineuses ou à liquide clair. Encycl Med Chir, Paris, 12, 6041, A30

Migueres J, Jover A, Krempf M (1975b) Note sur les incidents et accidents de la biopsie pleurale à l'aiguille: l'ensemencement néoplasique de la paroi (à propos de 300 épanchements et 440 fonctions-biopsies) (a propos of 300 effusions and 440 puncture biopsies). Poumon-Coeur 31: 347-349

Migueres J, Jover A (1981) Indications du talcage de plèvre sous pleuroscopie au cours des pleurésies malignes récidivantes. A propos de 26 observations. Poumon-Coeur 37: 295-298

Millar JW, Hunter AM, Horne NW (1980) Intrapleural immunotherapy with Corynebacterium parvum in recurrent malignant pleural effusions. Thorax 35: 856-858

Miller JI, Hatcher CR JR (1978) Thoracoscopy: a useful tool in the diagnosis of thoracic disease. Ann Thorac Surg 26: 68-72

Miller KS, Sahn SA (1987a) On the use of chest tubes. Chest 92: 960

Miller KS, Sahn SA (1987b) Chest tubes. Indications, technique, management and complications. Chest 91: 258-264

Miserocchi G (1985) Pleural liquid pressure. In: Chretien J, Bignon J, Hirsch A (eds) The pleura in health and disease, Dekker, New York, pp 151-168

Morel PH, Spiliopoulos A, Megevand R (1984) Pneumothorax spontané idiopathique: notre expérience de la pleurodèse à la Tétracycline. Med Hyg 42: 2150-2154

Morino H, Sakurai M, Kitamura H (1977) "Pleuritis Carcinomatosa" due to microscopical metastasis in diaphragm of cervical cancer. Report of a case. Med J Osaka Univ 28: 49-55

Mortenson RL, Kvale PA, Lewis J, Groux N (1987) Tetracycline pleurodesis in recurrent pneumothorax of benign etiology. Am Rev Respir Dis 135: A57

Muir JF, Defouilloy C, Ndarurinze S, Hermant A, Quequet PM, Broussier PM, Aubry P, Desablens B (1987a) Utilisation de la doxycycline intrapleurale par lavage-drainage dans les épanchements récidivants d'origine néoplasique. Rev Mal Resp 4: 29-33

Muir JF, Cerisel F, Defouilloy C, Broussier PM, Hermant A, Aubry P, Noarurinze S, Botto JM, Arlati S (1987b) Pleural drainage with talc vs Doxycycline in the control of malignant pleural effusions. Am Rev Respir Dis 135: A

Myers JA (1954) Simple spontaneous pneumothorax. Dis Chest 26: 420-441

Nadjafi AS, Konietzko N, Cegla UH, Matthys H (1976) La biopsie chirurgicale pleuro-pulmonaire chez les malades à haut risque pulmonaire. Bronchopneumologie 26: 219-224

Nandi P (1980) Recurrent spontaneous pneumothorax; an effective method of talc poudrage. Chest 77: 493-495

Newhouse MT (1989) Thoracoscopy: diagnostic and therapeutic indications. Pneumologie 43: 48-52

Nico JP (1950) Le traitement actif des pneumothorax idiopathiques récidivants par la symphyse pleurale provoquée (méthode au talc) à propos de 10 cas personnels. Poumon 6: 167-181

O'Neill W, Spurr C, Muss H, Richards F, White D, Cooper MR (1980) A prospective study of chest tube drainage and Tetracycline (TCN) sclerosis versus chest tube drainage alone in the treatment of malignant pleural effusion. Proc Am Soc Clin Oncol 21: 349

Oakes DD, Sherck JP, Brodsky JB, Mark JB (1984) Therapeutic thoracoscopy. J Thorac Cardiovasc Surg 87: 269-273

Ohata M, Suzuli H (1980) Pathogenesis of spontaneous pneumothorax: with special reference to the ultrastructure of emphysematous bullae. Chest 77: 771-776

Oldenburg FA JR, Newhouse MT (1979) Thoracoscopy. A safe, accurate diagnostic procedure using the rigid thoracoscope and local anesthesia. Chest 75: 45-50

Olivier AF (1982) Tetracycline pleurodesis for refractory pneumothorax among inoperable elderly surgical candidates. Chest 82: 512

Ostrowski MJ (1986) An assessment of the long-term results of controlling the reaccumulation of malignant effusions using intracavitary bleomycin. Cancer 57: 721-727

Ottow RT, Eggermont AM, Steller EP, Sugarbaker PH (1987) The requirements for successful immunotherapy of intraperitoneal cancer using interleukin-2 and lymphokine-activated killer cells. Cancer 60: 1465-1473

Palojoki A (1981) La thoracoscopie dans le diagnostic des affections pleurales. Poumon-Coeur 37: 63-65

Pearson FG, MAC Gregor DC (1966) Talc poudrage for malignant pleural effusion. J Thorac. Cardiovasc. Surg 51: 732-738

Pepper JR (1978) Thoracoscopy in the diagnosis of pleural effusions and tumours. Brist J Dis Chest 72: 74-75

Pizzocaro G, Ravasi GL, Bozzetti F, Vaglini M, Lamonica G (1973). L'intalcamento del cavo pleurico nel trattamento dei versamenti neoplastici recidivanti. Tumori 59: 287-294

Prorok J, Nealon TF (1968) Pleural symphysis by talc poudrage in the treatment of malignant pleural effusion. Bull Soc Int Chir 6: 630-636

Quetglas FS, Velasquez AS, Pujol JL (1985) La toracoscopia. Jarpyo, Madrid

Rambaldi A, Introna M, Colotta F, Landolfo S, Colombo N, Mangioni C, Mantovani A (1985) Intraperitoneal administration of interferon B in ovarian cancer patients. Cancer 56: 294-301

Ratzer ER, Pool JL, Melamed MR (1967) Pleural Mesotheliomas: clinical experiences with thirty-seven patients. Am J Roentgenol 99: 863-880

Reid L (1967) Thc pathology of emphysema. Lloyd Luke, London

Renault P (1978) Diagnostic étiologique des pleurésies à liquide clair par le cytodiagnostic et par les biopsies de plèvre. Rev Prat 28: 2077-2092

Research Committee of the British Thoracic Association and the Medical Research Council Pneumoconiosis Unit (1979) A survey of the long-term effects of talc and Kaolin pleurodesis. Br J Dis Chest 73: 285-288

Rinaldo JE, Owens GR, Rogers RM (1983) Adult respiratory distress syndrome following intrapleural instillation of talc. J Thorac Cardiovasc Surg 85: 523-526

Rioseco A (1980) More about NaOH in the management of malignant pleural effusions. Chest 77: 813

Roche G, Delanoe Y, Moayer N (1963) Talcage de la plèvre sous pleuroscopie. Résultats, indications, technique (A propos de 14 observations). J Fr Med Chir Thorac 17: 677-692

Roche G (1965) Le traitement local des pneumothorax spontanés. Poumon-Coeur 21: 177-195

Rodgers BM, Talbert JL (1976) Thoracoscopy for diagnosis of intrathoracic lesions in children. J Pediat Surg 11: 703-708

Rodgers BM (1979a) Thoracoscopy in childhood malignancy. J Flo Med Assoc 66: 620-622

Rodgers BM, Moazam F, Talbert JL (1979b) Thoracoscopy. Early diagnosis of interstitial pneumonitis in the immunologically suppressed child. Chest 75: 126-130

Rodgers BM (1981) Thoracoscopy in children. Poumon-Coeur 37: 301-306

Rossi GA, Felletti R, Balbi B, Sacco O, Cosulich E, Risso A, Melioli G, Ravazzoni C (1987) Symptomatic treatment of recurrent malignant pleural effusions with intrapleurally administered Corynebacterium parvum. Am Rev Respir Dis 135: 885-890

Rubinson RM, Bolooki H (1972) Intrapleural tetracycline for control of maligant pleural effusion: a preliminary report. South Med J 65: 847-849

Ruckley CV, Cormack JM (1966) The management of spontaneous pneumothorax. Thorax 21: 139-144

Rusch VW, Mountain C (1987) Thoracoscopy under regional anesthesia for the diagnosis and management of pleural disease. Am J Surg 154: 274-278

Sacco F (1952) Indicazioni dell'endoscopia pleurica nella diagnosi delle malattie toraciche. Minerva Med 43: 390-396

Sahn SA, Good JT (1981) The effect of common sclerosing agents on the rabbit pleural space. Am Rev Respir Dis 124: 65

Sahn SA (1988) The pleura. Am Rev Respir Dis 138: 184-234

Salyer WR, Eggleston JC, Erozan YS (1975) Efficacy of pleural needle biopsy and pleural fluid cytopathology in the diagnosis of malignant neoplasm involving the pleura. Chest 67: 536-539

Sattler A (1937) Zur Behandlung des Spontanpneumothorax mit besonderer Berücksichtigung der Thorakoskopie. Beitr Klin Tuberk 89: 395-408

Sattler A (1961) La biopsie pleurale. Résultats et rôle pratique. Symposium Ciba 9: 109-122

Sattler A (1966) Die Bedeutung der Endoskopie und Biopsie des Coeloms für medizinische Disziplinen. Wien Med Wschr 116: 439-445

Sattler A (1981) La thoracoscopie: intérêt thérapeutique dans les syndromes pleuro-pulmonaires d'urgence et intérêt diagnostique. Poumon-Coeur 37: 265-267

Scarbonchi J, Boutin C, Cargnino P, Scarbonchi-Efimief T (1981) Le talcage pleural dans les pleurésies cancéreuses. Poumon-Coeur, 37: 283-289

Scerbo J, Keltz H, Stone DJ (1971) A prospective study of closed pleural biopsy. JAMA 218: 377-380

Sebastien P (1982) La biométrologie des fibres inhalées. Dissertation University of Paris XII

Seitz B, Delpierre S, Choux R, Lama A, Boutin C (1989) Etude experimentale des effets pleuraux de la pulvérisation, sous contrôle thoracoscopique, d'une colle de fibrine (Tissucol). Rev Mal Resp 6: 537-542

Senigaglia P, Marchetti GP, Foccoli PF, Milano S, DI Fabio D, Tassi GF (1987) La terapia sinfisaria con tetraciclina nel pneumotorace spontaneo. In: Bergonzini R, Favagrosso GM, Malavisa D (eds) Aggiornamenti di radiologia toracica. APC-Sirmn, Brescia, vol VII, pp. 269-270

Senno A, Moallem S, Quijano ER, Adeyemo A, Clauss RH (1974) Thoracoscopy with the fiberoptic bronchoscope. A simple method in diagnosing pleuropulmonary diseases. J Thorac Cardiovasc Surg 67: 606-611

Senno A, Moallem S, Quijano ER, Tan BY, Clauss RH (1975) Fiberoptic thoracoscopy. NY J Med 75: 51-56

Shedbalkar AR, Head JM, Head LR, Murphy DJ, Mason JH (1971). Evaluation of talc pleural symphysis in management of malignant pleural effusion. J Thorac Cardiovasc Surg 61: 492-497

Sherman S, Grady KJ, Seidman JC (1987) Clinical experience with tetracycline pleurodesis of malignant pleural effusions. Southern Med J 80: 716-719

Sherman S (1988) Optimum anesthesia with intrapleural Lidocaïne during chemical pleurodesis with Tetracycline. Chest 93: 533-537

Sison BS, Weiss W (1962) Needle biopsy of the parietal pleura in patients with pleural effusion. Br Med J 5300: 298

Smith WG, Rothwel PG (1962) Treatment of spontaneous pneumothorax. Thorax 17: 342-349

Sorensen PG, Svendsen TL, Enk B (1984) Treatment of malignant pleural effusion with drainage. With and without instillation of talc. Eur J Respir Dis 65: 131-135

Spiegel M, Benesch J, Siebenmann R (1983) Thorakoskopische Pleurodeses bei spontanan Pneumothorax. Prax Klin Pneumol 37: 976-978

Stanek RG, Wilson JL, Rogers WL (1961) Spontaneous Pneumothorax: A review of 71 cases. Dis Chest 40: 391-396

Steele JD (1947) Production of pleural adhesions for therapeutic purposes. Am Rev Tub 56: 299-302

Stradling P, Poole G (1966) Conservative management of spontaneous pneumothorax. Thorax 21: 145-149

Swierenga J, Wagenaar JP, Bergstein PG (1974) The value of thoracoscopy in the diagnosis and treatment of diseases affecting the pleura and lung. Pneumologie 151: 11-18

Swierenga J (1977) Atlas of thoracoscopy. Boehringer, Ingelheim

Szule P (1989) Diagnostik des tuberkulösen pleuraergusses. Pneumologie 43: 66-68

Takeno Y (1978) Un nouveau traitement du pneumothorax spontané par nébulisation d'une colle liquide sous contrôle thoracoscopique. Broncho-Pneumol 28: 19-28

Tandon RK (1966) The significance of pleural effusions associated with bronchial carcinoma. Br J Dis Chest 60: 49-53

Taryle DA, Lakshminarayan S, Sahn SA (1976) Pleural Mesothelioma: an analysis of 18 cases and review of the literature. Medicine (Baltimore) 55: 153-162

Tassi GF (1983) Intrapleural tetracycline for recurrent pneumothorax. Chest 83: 836

Thomas PA, Gebauer PW (1958) Pleurectomy for recurrent spontaneous pneumothorax. J Thoracic Surg 35: 111-117

Thorsrud GK (1965) Pleural reaction to irritants. Acta Chir Scand 335: 11-25

Titscher R, Hatzenberger H (1974) Die Bedeutung der Pleuroskopie in der Differentialdiagnose der tuberkulösen Pleuritis exsudativa. Prax Pneumol 28: 562-565

Todd TRJ, Delarue NC, Ilves R, Pearson FG, Cooper JD (1980). Talc poudrage for malignant pleural effusion. Chest 78: 542-543

Toomes H, Linder A (1989) Thorakoskopische sympathektomie bei hyperhidrosis. Pneumologie 43: 107-108

Touraine R (1960a) Les aspects pleuroscopiques des pleurésies cancéreuses. Lyon Med 92: 1581-1593

Touraine R (1960b) La pleuroscopie dans le diagnostic des pleurésies cancéreuses. J Fr Med Chir Thorac 6: 735-744

Touraine R (1962) La pleuroscopie dans le diagnostic des épanchements pleuraux. Rev Prat 12: 1805-1808

Touraine R (1965) La pleuroscopie. Rev Prat 15: 547-552

Tribble CG, Selden RF, Rodgers BM (1986) Talc poudrage in the treatment of spontaneous pneumothoraces in patients with cystic fibrosis. Ann Surg 204: 677-680

Triol JH, Conston AS, Chandler SV (1984) Malignant mesothelioma. Cytopathology of 75 cases seen in a New Jersey community hospital. Acta Cytol (Baltimore) 28: 37-45

Vanderschueren RG (1981a) Le talcage pleural dans le pneumothorax spontané. Poumon-Coeur 37: 273-276

Vanderschueren RG (1981b) Thoracoscopie sous anesthésie locale. Poumon-Coeur 37: 21-23

Velardocchio JM, Boutin C, Irisson M (1984) La pression pleurale au cours des ponctions évacuatrices pour pleurésie néoplasique. Bull Eur Physiopathol Respir 20: 61-64

Verreault J, Lepage S, Bisson G, Plante A (1986) Ascites and right pleural effusion: demonstration of a peritoneo-pleural communication. J Nucl Med 27: 1706-1709

Viallat JR, Tubiana N, Boutin C, Farisse P, Lejeune C, Carcassonne Y (1986) Pleurésies des hémopathies: intérêt du talcage thoracoscopique. Rev Pneum Clin 42: 274-278

Viallat JR, Tubiana N, Boutin C, Farisse P, Lejeune C, Carcassone Y (1986) Talcage thoracoscopique des pleurésies des hémopathies. Nlle Rev Fr Hemato 28: 381-385

Viard H, Favre JP, Penin M (1984) Traitement chirurgical du pneumothorax spontané idiopathique. Lyon Chir 80: 301-302

Viskum K, Enk B (1981) Complications of thoracoscopy. Poumon-Coeur 37: 25-28

Viskum K (1989a) Contraindications and complications to thoracoscopy. Pneumologie 43: 55-57

Viskum K, Lange P, Mortensen J (1989b) Long term sequelae after talc pleurodesis for spontaneous pneumothorax. Pneumologie 43: 105-106

Voellmy W (1981) Résultats diagnostiques de la thoracoscopie dans les affections du poumon et de la plèvre. Poumon-Coeur 37: 67-73

Wagenaar JPM (1970) Do zogenaamde idiopathische spontane pneumothorax. Thesis, Leiden

Wagner JC, Berry G, Cooke TJ, Hill RJ, Pooley FD, Skidmore JW (1977) In: Inhaled particles. Walton WH (eds) Animal experiments with talc. Pergamon, Oxford, vol IV, pp 647-654

Wall CP, Gaensler EA, Carrington CB, Hayes JA (1981) Comparison of transbronchial and open biopsies in chronic infiltrative lung diseases. Am Rev Respir Dis 123: 280–285

Wallach HW (1975) Intrapleural tetracycline for malignant pleural effusions. Chest 68: 510–512

Webb HE, Oaten SW, Pike CP (1978) Treatment of malignant ascitic and pleural effusions with Corynebacterium parvum. Br Med J 1: 338–340

Weichselbaum R, Marck A, Hellman S (1977) Pathogenesis of pleural effusion in carcinoma of the breast. Int J Radiat Oncol Biol Phys 2: 963–965

Weimar W, Bantje TA, Bron AC, Hilvering C, Bolhuis RLH, Schellekens H (1981) Interferon therapy for pleural mesothelioma. In: De Maeyer E, Galasso G, Schellekens H (eds) The biology of interferon system. Elsevier Biomedical, Amsterdam

Weissberg D, Kaufman M, Zurkowski Z (1980a) Pleuroscopy in patients with pleural effusion and pleural masses. Ann Thorac Surg 29: 205–208

Weissberg D, Kaufman M (1980b) Diagnostic and therapeutic pleuroscopy. Experience with 127 patients. Chest 78: 732–735

Weissberg D (1981a) Pleuroscopy in empyema: is it ever necessary? Poumon-Coeur 37: 269–272

Weissberg D (1981b) Talc pleurodesis: a controversial issue. Poumon-Coeur 37: 291–294

Weissberg D, Kaufman M, Schwecher I (1981c) Pleuroscopy in clinical evaluation and staging of lung cancer. Poumon-Coeur 37: 241–243

Werdermann K, Greschuchna D, Maassen W (1974) Ergebnisse chirurgischer Lungen- und Pleurabiopsien. Thoraxchirurgie 22: 453–456

Wetzer K, Schilling W, Wenzel D, Scheuler D (1980) Die thorakoskopische Lungenbiopsie. Z Erkrank. Atem-Org 155: 82–88

Whitcomb ME, Schwartz MI (1971) Pleural effusion complicating intensive mediastinal radiation therapy. Am Rev Respir Dis 103: 100–107

Whitwell F, Rawcliffe RM (1971) Diffuse malignant pleural mesothelioma and asbestos exposure. Thorax 26: 6–22

Wied U, Andersen K, Schultz A, Rasmussen E, Watt-Boolsen S (1981) Silver nitrate pleurodesis in spontaneous pneumothorax. Scand J Thor Cardiovasc Surg 15: 305–307

Wied U, Halkier E, Hoeier-Madsen K, Plucnar B, Rasmussen E, Sparup J (1983) Tetracycline versus silver nitrate pleurodesis in spontaneous pneumothorax. J Cardiovasc Surg 86: 591–593

Wieser O, Wieser CO (1989) Indikationen zur thorakoskopie beim sekundären spontanpneumothorax. Pneumologie 43: 92–95

Wihlm JM, Roeslin N, Morand G, Pauli G, Witz JP (1981) Résultats comparés de la ponction, de la biopsie à l'aiguille, de la pleuroscopie et de la thoracotomie dans le diagnostic des pleurésies chroniques. Poumon-Coeur 37: 57–60

Wittmoser R (1984) Possibilities of using sympathectomy for treatment of pain syndromes. Appl Neurophysiol 47: 203–207

R Wolf GmbH (1979) 1879–1979 – 100 Jahre Cystoskopie. Wolf, Knittlingen

Wooten SA, Strange C, Barbarash R, Sahn SA (1987) Pharmacokinetics of tetracycline and lidocaine following intrapleural instillation. Am Rev Respir Dis 135: A245

Youmans CR, Delano WR, Minn MR, Derrick J (1970) Surgical management of spontaneous pneumothorax by bleb ligation and pleural dry sponge abrasion. Am J Surg 120: 644–648

Zaloznik AJ, Oswald SG, Langin M (1983) Intrapleural Tetracycline in malignant pleural effusions. A randomized study. Cancer 51: 752–755

Subject Index